THE PUERTO RICANS

VIKING FUND PUBLICATIONS IN ANTHROPOLOGY

Number Fifty-one   Colin M. Turnbull, *Editor*

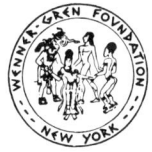

THE PUERTO RICANS
Culture Change and Language Deviance

RUBY ROHRLICH LEAVITT

Published for the Wenner-Gren Foundation for Anthropological Research Inc.

THE UNIVERSITY OF ARIZONA PRESS   TUCSON, ARIZONA

About the Author . . .

RUBY LEAVITT's Puerto Rican investigations sprang from an unusual merger of two disciplines from her own background—speech pathology, her former field of specialization, and anthropology—a latter-day field of interest. Her focus on Puerto Rico as part of the Caribbean Islands and Latin America she has continued in collaboration with her students at the Borough of Manhattan Community College, studying the impact of New York City on immigrants from those areas. As of the 1970s also, Dr. Leavitt was one of a group of women anthropologists re-analyzing the roles and status of women crossculturally. She has contributed to such volumes as *Woman in Sexist Society* and *Toward an Anthropology of Women* as well as to several other books and periodicals concerned with the study of sociocultural systems.

THE UNIVERSITY OF ARIZONA PRESS

I.S.B.N. -0-8165-0457-1
L.C. No. 73-90914

To my mother, Elise Rohrlich

Contents

PART IV. STUTTERING AND STRESSES

List of Tables

PART I

PERSPECTIVES ON STUTTERING

CHAPTER 1

Introduction

Stuttering has been known in the Western world for millennia, but not until the nineteenth century did Western observers discover that some non-Western peoples did not stutter. In the twentieth century, a number of scholars began to examine the characteristics of the cultures in which stuttering prevailed and of those that had no stuttering, and to speculate about the relationships between stuttering and social systems (Bloodstein 1958, Johnson 1967, Morgenstern 1956, Sheehan 1958, Travis 1957, Van Riper 1954). The theories remained largely unsubstantiated, however, for research into the sociocultural bases of stuttering etiology has been sporadic.

Overview of the Study

To determine whether sociocultural factors are basic in stuttering etiology, I investigated the incidence of stuttering in a single ethnic group, Puerto Rican rural migrants, living in two different cultural milieus, San Juan and New York City, and compared the sociocultural variables in the lifeways of the migrants in the two cities.

For the relevant background data on stuttering, I investigated the worldwide prevalence of stuttering, stuttering in connection with bilingualism, the sociocultural factors accounting for the differences in male and female stuttering incidence, and for the differences in stuttering incidence in the several socioeconomic classes.

In order to ascertain the sociocultural characteristics associated with stuttering and nonstuttering societies, I compared each of three cultures that had a high incidence with each of three that had no stuttering. Also, I drew composite profiles of the stuttering societies as a group and of the nonstuttering societies as a group and used these profiles as a baseline against which I compared the dominant values of Puerto Rico and the United States, to determine which characteristics they shared with the stuttering and nonstuttering groups. I also investigated the cultural variations and similarities among the rural subcultures from which the Puerto Ricans migrate so that I could determine their values and life patterns before they were changed in the culture of poverty in San Juan and New York.

For a view of the cultural setting in New York, I analyzed changing American values about work, dominant and working-class patterns of child rearing, American theories and practices in regard to acculturation and assimilation, and New York as a city of immigrants. I also discussed the incentives for the migration of rural Puerto Ricans to New York, and the problem of Puerto Rican identity, both on the island and the mainland, as it relates to their acculturation in New York.

To arrive at the differences in the socioeconomic status of the migrants in San Juan and New York, I compared their lifeways in the two cities in terms of occupation, income, consumer practices, housing and neighborhood life, religion, health, marriage and the family. I paid particular attention to the education and upward mobility of second-generation Puerto Ricans, for I was centrally concerned with the stresses underlying the differences in stuttering incidence of this generation in San Juan and New York.

Finally, I analyzed the relationships between stuttering incidence and sociocultural variables among the migrants in San Juan and New York, and drew inferences from these relationships about stuttering as a deviant linguistic response to cultural and socioeconomic stress.

Purpose and Design

This study is an attempt to investigate the validity of the theory that stuttering is a deviant linguistic response to sociocultural stress. Integrating the disciplines of speech pathology and the social sciences, particularly anthropology, I ascertained the stuttering incidence of a single ethnic group, the Puerto Ricans, living in two different cultural milieus, San Juan and New York City, and examined the differences in their lifeways in the two cities, proceeding on the premise that significant differences in stuttering incidence in the two milieus could be due only to significant differences between the respective lifeways.

For convenience of identification, I designate non-Puerto Rican Americans as "Americans," and Americans of Puerto Rican descent as

"Puerto Ricans," whether they were born in Puerto Rico or on the United States mainland. For the purposes of this study, I follow the definition of a Puerto Rican used by the New York City Board of Education, *Special Census of School Population,* October 31, 1963: "One parent or both parents, or child, born in Puerto Rico, regardless of skin color."

The sample populations studied in San Juan and New York each consisted of about 10,000 Puerto Rican children in the public elementary schools. The children in the San Juan population, a cross-section of the public school enrollment, were mainly members of the lower socioeconomic classes, since the vast majority of the children in the middle and upper-income classes of San Juan attend private schools (G. Lewis 1963:464). The Puerto Rican children in the New York population were also, for the most part, members of the lower socioeconomic classes. "Even among persons living in the city's poverty areas, Puerto Ricans find themselves pretty close to the bottom" (Lissner 1968:29). Thus socioeconomic status was approximately matched in the two populations.

The San Juan sample was drawn from grades one through six in the public schools. The New York City sample was drawn from grades one through six in public schools with a majority of Puerto Rican pupils, and consisted of children who had lived on the mainland for a minimum of three years. The parents of the Puerto Rican children attending the public schools in both cities were primarily migrants from the rural areas of Puerto Rico. But about three-fourths of the Puerto Rican children in New York were born on the mainland,[1] and their cultural milieu differs considerably from that of the San Juan children.

Although the migrants suffer from low socioeconomic status in both San Juan and New York, acculturation in New York requires adaptation to a different physical environment and culture. Parents and children must learn another language when they enter the job market and the schools. Families in New York are separated from relatives by far greater geographical distances than are the migrants in San Juan. Intergenerational conflicts are exacerbated in New York when the children acquire the values of a culture which differs from that of their parents. Racial discrimination in New York is more open and widespread than in San Juan, and Commonwealth status is often more keenly experienced as subordinate in New York.

According to Beals (1959:7), "rural-urban acculturation and cross-cultural acculturation differ only in degree and do not represent sub-

---

[1]Personal communication, Bureau of Educational Research, Board of Education, City of New York, March 20, 1968.

stantially different processes of change." Assuming that the difference in degree would make acculturation in New York more stressful than urbanization in San Juan, I hypothesized that sociocultural stress evokes a significantly higher incidence of stuttering among the children of the Puerto Rican migrants in New York than in San Juan.

But that was not the case. I found the incidence of stuttering in the sample population of San Juan to be significantly greater than in the sample population of New York (below the 1 percent level of significance). This unexpected finding in no way changed the course of the investigation. In fact, it sharpened my curiosity and whetted even more my interest in discovering the source of the stresses relating to the different incidence of stuttering among the Puerto Ricans in each milieu.

CHAPTER 2

Stuttering: Overview and Theories

Because speech is the basic form of human communication, stuttering,[1] one of the most serious impediments to communication, is a source of considerable frustration, stress, and even agony. Stuttering is "the speech difficulty of a person who tries to speak not wisely but too well" (Bloodstein 1958:5). The stutterer "knows precisely what word he wants to say; he is simply unable for the moment to say it" because he is struggling "against an imagined obstacle" to the articulation of sounds and words. Stuttering is generally preceded by the "anxious anticipation of stuttering" and is the "habit of making elaborate preparations for speech on the assumption that it is a difficult and treacherous process." Shakespeare described the stutterer's dilemma: "I would thou couldst stammer, . . . as wine comes out of a narrow-mouthed bottle, either too much at once, or none at all" (*As You Like It,* III, ii).

As the operational definition of stuttering, I used Van Riper's description:

The flow of speech is broken by hesitations, stoppages, or repetitions and prolongations of the speech sounds. Fluency is interrupted by spasms, contortions, tremors, or abnormalities of phonation and respiration. It [stuttering] consists of moments of speech interruption of such frequency and abnormality as to attract attention, interfere with communication, and produce maladjustment. It is the speech behavior that has been labeled by others and accepted by its possessor as "stuttering" (1954:23).

---

[1]For the purposes of this study, no distinction is made between mild and severe forms of stuttering, and between the terms "stammering" and "stuttering."

Historical Overview

No one knows how long stuttering has afflicted the human race, for speech leaves no mark on the human bones and stone artifacts that the archaeologist finds. But the earliest historical mention of stuttering appears in the records of the ancient Egyptian civilizations (Fletcher 1928:1), and both Old and New Testaments refer to speech impediments that have been interpreted as stuttering.

When God commanded Moses to tell the Egyptian pharaoh to set the Israelites free, Moses, with the typical fear of the stutterer, tried to avoid the confrontation. He pleaded: "I am not eloquent . . . but I am slow of speech and of a slow tongue" (Exodus iv, 10–17).

The despair of the stutterer was inscribed on a small clay tablet found in the ruins of the Biblical town of Beth Shemish: "Oh God, cut through the backbone of my stammering" (Greene 1935:2240).

The prophet Isaiah predicted that in some halcyon future "the tongues of stammerers shall speak readily and plain" (Isaiah xxxii, 4).

And Jesus cured a man of a speech defect that has been construed as stuttering: "And they bring unto Him one that was deaf and had an impediment in his speech" (St. Mark vii, 32).

Among the ancient Greeks, Hippocrates, the father of medicine, attributed stuttering to chronic diarrhea. Before he became a noted orator, Demosthenes studied diction to cure his stuttering. Aristotle was probably the first to ascribe stuttering to malfunctioning of the tongue, and this remained the dominant theory of the etiology of stuttering for almost 2,000 years (Klingbeil 1939:115). Little more than a century ago it was believed that stuttering could be cured by surgery of the tongue. In 1841, 200 tongue operations were performed in France during a twelve-month period, and 300 in England within six months. In the United States the popularity of tongue surgery was much shorter lived (Wallace et al. 1954:416).

Although there are nonstuttering societies, stuttering in general is not a respecter of country, rank, virtue, or genius. Eminent men who stuttered include Charles I of England; the English writers, Charles Lamb and Somerset Maugham; the English scientist, Charles Darwin; the French poet, François de Malherbe; the Italian mathematician, Nicolo Fontana, known as "Tartaglia" or "the stutterer"; the German-Jewish philosopher, Moses Mendelssohn; the Canadian actor, Raymond Massey; the American speech pathologist, Wendell Johnson.

Attitudes toward people who stutter have ranged from revulsion and rejection to mockery. In Roman times, for example, "cages along the Appian Way held grotesque human disabilities, including 'Balbus Blaesus,' the stutterer, who would attempt to talk when a coin was flung through the bars" (Van Riper 1954:4).

It was not until the eighteenth century Enlightenment that compassion became a more typical reaction toward the handicapped. But the scientific investigation of the causes of stuttering had to wait for the development of such modern sciences as physiology, psychology, speech pathology, linguistics, anthropology, and sociology, when stuttering came to be viewed as a problem and a challenge.

Theories about Stuttering Etiology

Modern scientific research into the etiology of stuttering began in the nineteenth century, when it was concerned primarily with physiological causes. In the twentieth century, the research became much more extensive and centered about psychological factors. Increasingly, anthropological and sociological concepts have been applied, adding new dimensions to the investigations.

NEUROPHYSIOLOGICAL THEORIES

During the first half of the nineteenth century, stuttering was the domain of the medical profession and causes were attributed mainly to physiological factors. Neurophysiological, organic, and genetic theories continued to be influential in the twentieth century, and increasingly refined studies of stuttering have been done in relation to the action of the cerebral hemispheres and the cortex of the brain, cardiovascular patterns, blood pressure, basal metabolism, blood-sugar ratings, allergies, motor proficiency, multiple births, and laterality.

A review of 150 studies, however, showed a lack of correlation between stuttering and biochemical or physiological factors. "An agent in the form of an inner condition . . . is still as distant from discovery as it was 4000 years ago" (Hill 1944:245–61, 289–327). Moreover, even those speech pathologists who regard neurophysiological factors as primary now also consider psychological and social influences in the etiology and/or persistence of stuttering (Karlin, Karlin and Gurren 1965).

PSYCHOLOGICAL THEORIES

Psychological theories about stuttering came to the fore during the latter half of the nineteenth century. Freud's published writings contain very few references to stuttering, but a number of physicians of the Freudian school characterized the defect as a psychoneurosis, to be treated mainly by psychoanalysis. A survey of the research, however, revealed "no evidence that the etiology of stuttering is rooted in gross psychological pathology" (Goodstein and Dahlstrom 1956:370) of either the parents of stutterers or of stutterers themselves. Stutterers do not appear to be severely maladjusted when compared with psychotic people, but are usually "somewhat more anxious, tense and socially withdrawn" when compared with individuals judged to be normal:

it is impossible to conclude from these studies whether these problems were etiological to the development of stuttering, or developed as a consequence of the social reaction to the stutterer (Goodstein 1958:371).

All the research points to anxiety as a concomitant of stuttering. "Those situations that allow for reduced anxiety about stuttering will usually allow for a reduction in stuttering" (Adler 1961:39).

Influenced by behavioral learning theories, a number of speech pathologists began to explain the onset and persistence of stuttering as learned behavior. Foremost was Wendell Johnson, who in the 1930s set forth the "general interaction" or "diagnosogenic" or semantic theory about the etiology of stuttering. Johnson hypothesized that stuttering arises as a problem when a listener, usually a parent, evaluates a child's hesitations and repetitions as stuttering and reacts to them with concern and disapproval. The child reacts to this concern by speaking more disfluently. He becomes sensitive to his own speech, as well as to the negative evaluation, and this sensitivity interferes with the automaticity of his speech. A nonfluent speaker whose speech is accepted as being within the range of normal speech does not have the problem of stuttering. The question is, what cultural factors lead to the evaluation of speech as either "stuttering" or "normal."

LINGUISTIC THEORIES AND STUTTERING

Repetition or Reduplication. In a study of 150 stuttering and 150 nonstuttering children, only the parents of the stuttering children evaluated their children as stutterers when they repeated sounds, syllables and words. Despite the fact that all the children in the study spoke with about the same number and kinds of disfluencies, "the parents of the so-called stutterers judged that their children were stuttering, but the parents of the nonstuttering children judged that their children were speaking normally for their age and level of development" (Johnson 1967:232).

According to anthropologists and speech pathologists, repetition and reduplication are universal speech phenomena, especially among babies and young children. Sapir wrote that "nothing is more natural than the prevalence of reduplication . . . the repetition of all or part of the radical element" (1921:79). Casagrande noted "the universality of reduplication" in the baby words of all languages, written and oral (1964:247). The Manus of the Admiralty Islands used repetition to teach children how to speak. Mead observed that "this random affection for repetitiousness makes an excellent atmosphere in which the child acquires facility in speech" (1930:37). The outstanding speech characteristic of the two-year-old child appears to be an "almost compulsive" repetitiveness. He "seems to be consolidating the past six months' progress, and repeats words and phrases as though fascinated" (Metraux 1950:51).

The Sapir-Whorf Hypothesis. The anthropologist Edward Sapir made important contributions to the theories about the role of language in human societies. He pointed out that "vocabulary is the very sensitive index of the culture of a people" (1966a:36), and hypothesized that language mediated the objective and social worlds for human beings:

the "real world" is to a large extent unconsciously built up on the language habits of the group. No two languages are ever sufficiently similar to be considered as presenting the same social reality (Sapir 1966b:69).

To this hypothesis Whorf added his concept of linguistic relativity, stating in part that the world view of a society stemmed from its language patterns, which codified the consensus or agreement of the speech community.

The agreement is, of course, an implicit and unstated one, but its terms are absolutely obligatory: we cannot talk at all except by subscribing to the organization and classification of data which the agreement decrees (1964:107).

Influenced by the Sapir-Whorf hypothesis, Johnson postulated that the presence of words for stuttering in a lexicon indicated a cultural predisposition to evaluate certain speech patterns as stuttering. The labeling of certain kinds of speech behavior as "stuttering" reflects cultural perceptions and judgments which "have been influenced by the patterns of selection and organization characteristic of our respective languages" (Johnson 1958:xiii).

Speech pathologists have been applying the findings of anthropology and linguistics for almost half a century. But not until the 1960s did the linguists begin to consider the importance which speech pathologies might hold for a general theory of language (Diebold 1965). This followed the birth of the new subdiscipline of pyscholinguistics, with its express purpose of studying speech behavior: "how we learn to speak, the relations between speaking and thinking, and deviations in speech behavior like stuttering and aphasia" (A. G. Smith 1966:3). In a recent survey of psycholinguistic research, it was noted with satisfaction,

that the study of speech pathologies is attracting ever more attention by linguists and psycholinguists who are discovering—even in the therapists' rules for treatment—hitherto overlooked insights into the nature of language (Diebold 1965:252).

CULTURE AND STUTTERING

More than a century ago James Hunt, an early British anthropologist, linked speech disorders with cultural factors when he noted the absence of such disorders among preliterate peoples.

All travellers who have long resided among uncultivated nations and whose authority is of any weight maintain that they have never met with any savages laboring under an impediment of speech. . . . Their freedom from mental anxieties and nervous debility . . . offers the best explanation of the alleged fact (1861:39).

Wendell Johnson was the speech pathologist who pioneered the investigation of stuttering among such "uncultivated nations" as the North American Indians. In this research, scholars were concerned not only with the incidence of stuttering but also with speech patterns and cultural attitudes toward speech and child rearing. They had available a corpus of anthropological theory and data, including ethnographies of individual cultures which made possible cross-cultural comparisons.

A number of speech pathologists and psychologists now associate stuttering with cultural and social variables. According to Johnson, a child may learn to stutter in a society that places a very high premium on speech fluency, for in such a society a child hesitates to hesitate and fears to repeat. Morgenstern (1953) found that the incidence of stuttering was highly correlated with the cultural stigmatization of certain kinds of speech as stuttering.

Bloodstein (1959) concluded that the prevalence of stuttering reflected a culture that was competitive, intolerant of inadequate performance, and very strongly emphasized the goals of status and prestige. In Euro-American cultures, the much higher stuttering incidence among males than females is due to the much greater emphasis on competition and achievement for males than for females, according to Sheehan (1958: 163). Morgenstern's research also indicated that "socioeconomic conditions have an important bearing on stammering incidence" (1953:59).

Sheehan pointed out that in Western industrialized nations, time pressure, a fundamental factor in stuttering, mediated interpersonal relations, particularly between superordinates and subordinates, and created anxiety, guilt, and conflicts, which are fertile grounds for the development of stuttering (1958:143–45). American children, according to Van Riper (1954:349), were pressed to acquire fluent speech at too early an age and at the same time that many prohibitions were imposed on them. Anxiety, fear, and shame accompany many kinds of behavior in the United States, said Travis (1957:918–25), and the attempt to cope with these emotions affects all responses, including speech.

CHAPTER 3

Related Literature

To provide the relevant background on stuttering, this section of the chapter deals with the incidence of stuttering on a worldwide basis, bilingualism and stuttering, the differences between male and female stuttering incidence cross-culturally and subculturally, and stuttering incidence in the several socioeconomic classes.

Incidence and Prevalence of Stuttering

The incidence and prevalence of stuttering in various cultures throughout the world demonstrate the range from no stuttering to high incidence.

In the United States the incidence of stuttering is estimated to range from about 0.6 to 1 percent (Johnson 1967:244). "The largest single group of handicapped children in the nation's schools today," 2.5 million children, have serious speech and language disorders. About "1 percent . . . possess a rhythm disorder which is commonly called stuttering" (Marge 1965:24).

Stuttering incidence is reported to be slightly less than 1 percent in England, Denmark, Hungary, Belgium, and other European countries (Bloodstein 1958:13). But in one European subculture, the Hebridean Island of North Uist, only two adult stutterers were found in a population of 2,500 people (Morgenstern 1953:59).

Surveys in India, Ghana and South Africa also show an incidence of about 1 percent (Andrews and Harris 1964:8), and stuttering is prevalent in China and Japan. In West Africa only the Hausa of northern Nigeria have no stuttering. "Of all the peoples who inhabited the west coast of Africa—from the British Cameroons to Nigeria, the Gold Coast and Sierra Leone—not one was found who do not stammer—except the Hausa" (Morgenstern 1953:242).

Among the Indians of North America the range is from no stuttering to a high incidence. Since the lexicons of the nonstuttering societies generally have no words for stuttering, it is assumed that stuttering is prevalent among cultures that have words for it. Sapir (1959) found a high incidence among the Nootka of Vancouver Island who used several words for stuttering, and Kroeber (1960) noted that the Yurok of northwest California had several words for stuttering. The Navajo of Arizona and New Mexico have a moderate incidence (Bullen 1945:3–7), and the Ute of Utah and Colorado have no stuttering (Johnson 1944).

The Polynesians are a "low-incidence" people (Lemert 1962). The following peoples neither stutter nor have words for stuttering in their languages: 2,500 Wapishianas, 1,100 Patamonas, and 1,500 Akawaio in Guyana; the Kelabits of West Borneo; about 60,000 Negritos, Semoi and aboriginal Malays in Malaya, speaking some 16 languages; about 20,000 laborers and their families in Assam, India, including the Sonthals, Bhuyana, and Gatwas from Behar, and the Tantis from Orissa, speaking many dialects; the Garia of New Guinea (Morgenstern 1953:239–240); seven New Guinea tribes, with different cultures, consisting of about 6,000 people, studied by Mead; the Australian aborigines studied by Warner; 250 Eskimos in Northwest Greenland studied by Eckblaw (Bullen 1945:7–10).

Bilingualism and Stuttering

Psycholinguistic research in bilingualism is concerned with the possible interference by an established language in the learning of a second one. In determining the cultural factors that interfere with the learning of a second language, however, the linguist needs the help of the anthropologist, who views language contact within the total framework of culture contact, "and language interference as a facet of cultural diffusion and acculturation. The linguist who makes theories about language influence but neglects to account for the sociocultural setting of the language contact leaves his study suspended . . . in mid-air" (Weinreich 1961:380). On the other hand, anthropologists must explore linguistic aspects as an index of the total acculturative process.

According to Lambert, an authority on bilingualism among French and English speakers in Canada, learning a second language successfully depends on "an appropriate attitudinal orientation toward the second language." Because bilingual speakers usually develop greater cognitive flexibility, they "are *far* superior to monolinguals on both verbal and non-verbal tests of intelligence" (Diebold 1965:251–252).

Few studies connect bilingualism with stuttering. "Some observers report cases of stuttering or blockage in infants exposed to two languages before one has been completely learned. . . . But there is no evidence of causal correlation" (Haugen 1961:398).

In 1937, a study was conducted to determine the influence of bilingualism on the incidence of stuttering in the public schools of East Chicago, Indiana, an industrial area with many foreign-born residents who were drastically affected by the economic depression of the 1930s. Among 4,800 students aged four to seven, the incidence of stuttering was 2.8 percent for the bilingual white children, compared with 1.8 percent for the white children who spoke only English.

We cannot be certain . . . that the difference is due solely to the factor of bilingualism. It may be due to the economic insecurity and emotional instability found in many foreign homes as a result of the recent depression (Travis, Johnson and Shover 1937:189).

Although a stuttering incidence of 3.76 percent was found among the blacks in East Chicago, the investigators did not suggest that the even greater economic insecurity of the blacks could account for their higher stuttering incidence.

Both peoples who do not stutter and those who have a high incidence of stuttering are bilingual. There was no stuttering among the bilingual Scottish children of North Uist in the Hebrides, or among the bilingual Ute of Colorado and Utah, or among the multilingual Murngin of Australia. But the multilingual Indians of the Northwest Pacific Coast had a high stuttering incidence. A survey of speech defects in the New York City public schools showed a stuttering incidence of 0.65 percent among the bilingual Puerto Ricans, compared with 1.05 percent among the monolingual blacks (Rivers 1964). Thus, bilingualism *per se* does not appear to be a factor in the etiology of stuttering.

Sex Ratio and Stuttering

In the United States, the higher incidence of all types of speech disorders among males, from early childhood on, led some speech pathologists to conclude that males were biologically more vulnerable than females to deviations in speech and language. But when the cultural significance of stuttering was recognized, the higher male incidence began to be viewed as evidence of the greater social demands on the male.

According to Ruth Benedict, the discontinuities in the male role are inescapable because the dependence of the son is in such marked contrast to the protective role of the father. Some cultures lessen the discontinuities by emphasizing praise and approval instead of obedience, in the rearing of males. Other cultures minimize the strain of the transition to manhood by effecting it publicly and ceremoniously after intensive preparation. In the United States, where dominance-submission is a striking aspect of behavior, "an individual conditioned to one set of behavior in childhood must adopt the opposite as an adult" (Benedict 1950:415) without a formal *rite de passage* to absorb the psychological strain of the transition.

Schuell found that the sex ratios in the incidence of stuttering parallel those in various behavior problems reported by teachers, child welfare clinics and juvenile research institutes, and she concluded that the same social pressures underlie both the higher stuttering incidence and greater behavior problems among boys. Parents and teachers reward boys less and punish them more than girls for the same behavior because they assume that the more severe treatment of boys will make them stronger, more independent and self-controlled in the competitive situations they encounter as children and adults. At the same time, both sexes are required to be equally obedient and submissive. These attitudinal differences toward the sexes are all the more incongruous, according to Schuell, because the male child is biologically less sturdy than the female and slower to develop language abilities. Thus, she concluded, the social pressures that produce greater maladjustment among males also create a higher stuttering incidence among them (Schuell 1947:23–38).

The studies discussed below show a range of disparities between male and female incidence in the several socioeconomic classes in the United States and other societies. Among middle-class children in the United States, male incidence is significantly higher than female, but in some lower socioeconomic groups there is little or no difference. And in Japan female incidence is reported to be higher than male. Sex ratios range from 1:1 to 10:1, the average in the United States being about 4:1. These and all subsequent ratios are male to female.

In a speech survey covering 4,685 elementary school children in Holyoke, Massachusetts, in 1940–41, more boys than girls were found to have articulatory problems of all kinds, more than three-fourths of the serious cases were boys, and more pressure was placed on boys to become fluent. Among the stutterers the ratio was 5:1 (Mills and Streit 1942:161).

In the public elementary schools in the middle- and upper-class suburb of Great Neck, New York, 25 children out of a population of 4,504 were found to stutter, the incidence being 0.5 percent. The sex ratio was 22 boys to 3 girls, or 7.3:1.[1]

Eisenson (1966) reported that the incidence of stuttering and the sex ratio in four *kibbutzim* in Israel were about the same as in the United States, even though the Israeli children were brought up communally with their peers, and the same child-rearing methods were used with both sexes.

Several studies in the United States showed greater disparity in stuttering incidence between white boys and girls than between black boys and girls. In eight segregated elementary schools in Topeka, Kansas, the sex ratio among black stutterers was 3.6:1, but among white stutterers it was 9.24:1 (Waddle 1934). Among second-grade children in the parochial schools of Orleans parish in Louisiana, a statistically significant difference was found between white male and female stutterers, but not between black males and females. Also, the incidence of stuttering among black females was significantly higher than among the white females. Even though these schools contained a fairly large proportion of middle- and upper-class black families, they were more "matricentric" than the white families (Neely 1960).

In a study of predominantly black elementary schools in Nashville, Tennessee, a marked difference was found in the sex ratio among stutterers in "patriarchal" and "matriarchal" environments. The criterion for a "patriarchal" environment was the consistent presence of a stable, financially responsible male in the home; for the "matriarchal," the absence of such a male. In the "patriarchal" segment the ratio was 3.5:1; in the "matriarchal," 1.1:1.

The first part of the study surveyed an almost equal male-female population among both white and black children. The black ratio was 2.35:1, and the white ratio was 4.93:1, or more than double the black ratio. Again, proportionately more black females stuttered than white females.

The ratio of 3.5:1 in the black "patriarchal" segment approximated the expected sex ratio of 4:1 among stutterers in the United States. The ratio in the black "matriarchal" segment, 1.1:1, reflected either increased pressure on the female or decreased demands on the male.

The results of this study, therefore, would seem to go along with the hypothesis indicated by Johnson . . . that unequal environmental pressures placed

---

[1]Personal communication from Doris Cleary, Chairwoman, Speech and Hearing Services, Great Neck Public Schools, Great Neck, N.Y., December 13, 1967.

on the male might account for the commonly observed male favored sex ratio in the incidence of stuttering (Goldman 1967:80).

The implications of this theory for Japan, where more girls were reported to stutter than boys (Lemert 1962:6), are that the environmental pressures are heavier on the girls.

Socioeconomic Classes and Stuttering Incidence

The research shows that stuttering occurs in all classes, and while it is agreed that "socioeconomic conditions have an important bearing on stammering incidence" (Morgenstern 1953:59), the authorities disagree about which class has the higher incidence.

Johnson and his coworkers (1959) found that the highest incidence of stuttering occurred in the middle and upper classes. In one study, 80 percent of 50 stuttering children, and in another study, 70 percent of 150 stuttering children were in these strata. In a third study, which matched 126 stutterers with 252 nonstutterers for age, race, sex, and location, the parents of one-third of the stutterers were found to be in the three highest occupational categories compared with the parents of one-sixth of the nonstutterers (Johnson 1956:356).

Bloodstein (1958) associated a higher stuttering incidence with greater competitiveness and the imposition of complex behavioral standards on children, characteristic of American segments "which are socioeconomically the most upward-moving."

In a survey of about 30,000 school children in Scotland, Morgenstern found a significantly higher incidence of stuttering among children whose fathers were semiskilled workers, a significantly low incidence among children whose fathers were unskilled workers, and an expected incidence among children whose fathers had middle- and upper-class occupations. Morgenstern (1956) concluded that the higher incidence among the children of the semiskilled was a reaction to parental pressure to become able speakers as a way of improving their class status.

A number of studies, however, show that the highest incidence of stuttering occurs among the lowest socioeconomic strata. A survey of about 7,400 nine-to-eleven-year-old school children in Newcastle-upon-Tyne, England, revealed that many of the stutterers lived in an environment significantly marked by economic deprivation and social pathology, such as broken homes, a lack of parental care, and a complete dependence upon social agencies (Andrews and Harris 1964:33, 103).

The studies comparing stuttering incidence among black and white children in the United States show a higher incidence among the blacks who are more economically deprived.

Among 579 lower-class black children in the first three grades of Lincoln Parish, Louisiana, 24 percent were found to need professional attention out of 26.9 percent who had speech defects. According to the Mid-Century White House Conference, 10 percent of the national school population were speech defective, and 5 percent required professional help (Evans 1964).

In the Topeka, Kansas, elementary schools, the incidence of stuttering was 7.21 percent among the blacks and 4.11 percent among the whites (Waddle 1934). In East Chicago, Indiana, the stuttering incidence among black elementary school children was 3.76 percent, compared with 2.3 percent among the white children (Travis, Johnson and Shrover 1937). The Orleans Parish parochial schools study showed a stuttering incidence of 1.99 percent among black children and 0.83 percent among white children (Neely 1960). A study of speech defects in the elementary and junior high schools of New York City revealed an incidence of 1.05 percent among blacks, and 0.42 percent among "others" (Rivers 1964).

Thus, in competitive society that describes itself as "open," the higher stuttering incidence among those strata that are socioeconomically deprived *without* opportunity for upward mobility appears to derive from greater stress, frustration and anxiety than exist among strata that are permitted to move upward.

In sum, the related literature shows the prevalence of stuttering in the United States, Europe, the British Isles, India, Burma, China, Japan, Israel, South Africa, and West Africa. But within these countries exist subcultures that have no stuttering, such as the Scottish subculture of North Uist, the Ute Indians and an Eskimo group in North America, the Hausa of northern Nigeria, and various subcultures in India. Nor was stuttering found among most aboriginal cultures in New Guinea, Australia, Malaya, West Borneo, and Guyana. Bilingualism does not appear to be causally related to stuttering, since stuttering is absent among some bilingual peoples and prevalent among others.

The disparities between male and female stuttering incidence appear to be linked to both cultural and socioeconomic factors. Although stuttering is found among all socioeconomic classes in open, competitive societies, the incidence appears to be highest among those groups that are given the least opportunity for upward mobility.

Table 3.1—Stuttering and Nonstuttering Sociocultural Variables:

North America—The Kwakiutl and the Ute

	Kwakiutl (Stuttering)[1]	Ute (Nonstuttering)[2]
Ecology	favorable natural resources and leisure time permitted development of complex political, social, religious institutions and art forms	scarce natural resources led to incessant nomadism; subsistence easier with advent of horse
Social Structure	tribes of nobles, commoners, slaves; cooperative in preparing products for potlatch and waging war; intense interpersonal and intertribal competition	extended family basic, but bands important with advent of horse raiding, buffalo hunting; war and war honors not institutionalized; authority vested in elders
Social Goals	accumulation of titles, validated at potlatch, and of material property to gain rank and prestige	cooperative family, band life; wisdom, maturity; when higher subsistence level reached, property shared
Paths to Goals	primogeniture; advantageous marriage; shamanism; murder and war; conspicuous destruction of property; self-glorification through oratory and shaming of rivals	gradual accumulation of wisdom, maturity through experience; ability to deal with personal, group stress rewarded by religious leadership; secular leadership, reward for hunting skills
Religion	harsh and punitive gods; rivalry between men and gods; cannibalism a religious ritual	harmonious cosmos; religion a source of social cohesion, individual and group health, endurance of nomadism
Family Life	primogeniture led to sibling rivalry; intense competition for titles marked affinal relations	parents, chief economic producers and grandparents raised children; divorce common, easy
Valued Attributes	competitiveness, aggressiveness, achievement orientation, ego-strength, oratorical ability	cooperation, deference to elders, industriousness, sobriety, oratorical ability
Child Rearing	children introduced early into competitive potlatch pattern; physical punishment for failure to observe religious rules; boys emulated boastful, insulting oratory	children petted, indulged; joking relations permitted aggression toward adults; no physical punishment; discipline by mild ridicule, threats of supernatural

Table 3.1—(Continued)

	Kwakiutl (Stuttering)[1]	Ute (Nonstuttering)[2]
Speech Attitudes	preacculturation stuttering, words for stuttering, penalties for stuttering; oratory, a means to achievement and shaming rivals	no stuttering, no words for stuttering; infantile repetitions; diminutive, affectionate language; terms for different childhood stages; child always considered satisfactory speaker; speech unhurried, deliberate; oratorical ability important
Stresses	incessant striving for goals; constant fear of ridicule, failure; intolerance of linguistic, physical handicaps	incessant mobility; ubiqitous authority of elders; fear of ancestral ghosts

Stuttering and Nonstuttering Societies

In order to determine the cultural and socioeconomic traits associated with stuttering and nonstuttering societies, I compared, in Tables 3.1–3.3 below, paired stuttering and nonstuttering cultures: the Kwakiutl and the Ute in North America; the Ibo and the Hausa in Nigeria, West Africa; the Japanese and the Scots of the Hebrides. Thus, stuttering and nonstuttering societies coexist not only in the same broad culture areas, but the Japanese and the Scots are peoples in modern industrialized countries, at relatively similar levels of technological development. The values of the cultures in each pair are in vivid contrast.

Following Tables 3.1–3.3 are composite profiles of the stuttering societies as a group and of the nonstuttering societies as a group, which treat more fully the variables concerned with family life, child-rearing practices and speech patterns. I used these profiles in the final chapter as a baseline against which I compared the dominant values of Puerto Rico and the United States, to ascertain which characteristics they shared with the stuttering and nonstuttering societies.

The profiles of the stuttering and nonstuttering cultures show that

---

[1]Sources of information about the Kwakiutl and similar cultures on the Northwest Pacific Coast were: Benedict (1959), Goldman (1961), Lemert (1952, 1953), Mead (1961), Pettit (1946), Sapir (1959), Spencer et al. (1965), Stewart (1960).

[2]Sources of information about the Ute were: Johnson (1944), Opler (1940, 1959), Snidecor (1947), Spencer et al. (1965), Stewart (1960).

Table 3.2—Stuttering and Nonstuttering Sociocultural Variables:

West Africa—The Ibo and the Hausa

	The Ibo (Stuttering)[1]	The Hausa (Nonstuttering)[2]
Ecology and Occupations	5 million-plus population, rural and urban areas; Ibo spread out and incorporate other peoples and easily assimilate other cultures; disproportionately employed in industry and government	6 million-plus people; mainly farmers, but because of short rainy season, farmers also have other traditional occupations
Social-Political Structure	lineage, clan, village memberships carried over into cities, help adaptation to urban life; former intervillage warfare transformed into village competition for schools, etc.; open, competitive society, with achieved leadership	highly centralized, hierarchical, stable, conservative, traditional chiefdoms; leadership economic, social, political, re-inherited; market central to ligious life
Social Goals	for men: wives and children; titles, secular and religious leadership; traditional and modern occupations for men and women	for men: wives and children; variety of traditional occupations; authority vested in elders; for women: children and craft production
Paths to Goals	money, education, oratory, European equipment	kin and bond friendships; gift-giving
Religion	headhunting, cannibalism formerly associated with warfare, paganism; now, paganism combined with Christianity	Islam combined with paganism
Family Life	strong mother-child and sibling bonds; only men obtain divorce, but women's increasing economic independence lessening male authority; modern education for women raises bride-price: later marriage, decrease in polygyny, more consensual unions and prostitution	extended kin very important, especially for women; divorce easy for men and women; because of wife-seculsion, women do not engage in farm labor, but have personal income from crafts production
Valued Attributes	competitiveness, aggressiveness, achievement orientation, receptivity to change, oratorical ability	cooperation among kin and bond friends; generosity and gift giving; oratorical ability

Table 3.2—(Continued)

	The Ibo (Stuttering)[1]	The Hausa (Nonstuttering)[2]
Child Rearing	children indulged and school represents sharp discontinuity; girls, hardworking, early age; boys, little responsibility until puberty, but then must start making money for goals and obligations	joking relations permit agression against adults; boys punished by paternal uncle; young girls trade for mothers, aunts, in market; young children's associations tour countryside, unsupervised: institutionalized "sweethearting"; marriage, severe discontinuity for women
Speech Attitudes	preacculturation stuttering; stuttering, great social handicap; stutterers ridiculed; oratorical ability very important even before adolescence; primary school subjects in own language	stuttering among all West Africans except Hausa; no word for stuttering in Hausa dictionary; grave, deliberate speech admired; parents tolerant of linguistic variations among small children; primary school subjects in own language
Stresses	individual must achieve for self and group; incessant striving for money, prestige, position; family strains because of increased female economic independence	for women: wife-seclusion, male homosexuality and widespread prostitution, arranged marriages; for men and women: brittle marriages

although each group comprises societies in widely separated geographical areas, the cultures within each group share dominant values. But, as in the paired societies, the values of the two groups are in sharp contrast.

CULTURAL PROFILE OF THE STUTTERING SOCIETIES

The similarity of goals and values among the Kwakiutl, the Ibo, and the Japanese is in striking contrast with the differences in their socioeconomic and ecological environments. Out of the bountiful natural resources of the Kwakiutl, the Ibo land scarcity, and the self-contained Japanese islands come the same traits of competitiveness and aggressiveness, developed to achieve the same goals of rank and property.

---

[1]Sources of information about the Ibo were: Basden (1921), Morgenstern (1953), P. Ottenberg (1959), S. Ottenberg (1959).

[2]Sources of information about the Hausa were: Goode (1963), Greenberg (1960), Morgenstern (1953), S. Ottenberg (1959), M. Smith (1954).

Table 3.3—Stuttering and Nonstuttering Sociocultural Variables:

Japan and the Hebrides

	Japan (Stuttering)[1]	Hebrides (Nonstuttering)[2]
Ecology	self-contained islands; highly developed technology and art	island subculture; main occupations: farming, sheepherding, fishing
Social-Political Structure	hierarchical extended family; economic patronage links within democratic capitalism	closely knit extended family, community; British subculture
Social Goals	advancement of family line; individual must succeed for himself and family	maintenance of economy; migration, immigration
Paths to Goals	patronage network backs able individual; education; male adoption; marriage	education; hard work; cooperation; welfarism
Religion	Confucianism, Buddhism, Shinto, Bushido: ancestor worship; obedience; loyalty to superordinates	vestiges, Celtic Druid beliefs; Catholicism; Calvinism
Marriage and Family	marriages arranged; patriarchal, patrilocal, patrilineal; tension, female affinal kin; all females subordinate; male sibling rivalry	nuclear, within extended family; egalitarian conjugal relations; no moral stigma, marriage immediately preceding childbirth
Valued Attributes	for women: subordination, continual deference, males and elders; for men: competitiveness, aggressiveness, striving, achievement orientation, subordination, male elders	individualism within cooperative system; independence; egalitarianism; generosity; hospitality; humor; physical stamina for men and women
Child Rearing	children loved unconditionally; school entrance, sharp discontinuity—children represent family, must never shame it; every school child promoted, given prize, lest he lose face, commit suicide; highly competitive exams, every school level	children loved, indulged; physical punishment for serious infractions, home and school; children participate economically; no pressure for academic achievement, but many islanders are university honors scholars; one-room schools, most islands

Table 3.3—(Continued)

	Japan (Stuttering)[1]	Hebrides (Nonstuttering)[2]
Speech Attitudes	parents shamed if child speaks deviantly, late; mother pressured to correct stuttering; schools, magazines, offer stuttering treatment; stuttering, occupational, social handicap, especially for girls	children speak Gaelic until school entrance, English learned as second language; children learn to speak at own pace; no demand for linguistic precocity; oaths, blasphemy, common among adults; gossip widespread—outlet for stress from close living
Stresses	individual always responsible for family name; constant repression, anger and resentment, especially by women; family relations very difficult; intolerance of linguistic, physical defects	economy no longer viable, islands depopulating rapidly; strains created by very close family, community relations

In the three societies the individual is supported by the group and must therefore achieve for the group, but achievement depends on his own ability and aggressiveness, and the penalties for failure are harsh. Among the Japanese an incompetent son may be supplanted as his father's heir. Only by incessant striving is an Ibo able to achieve prestigious titles and the bride-price for a wife. The Kwakiutl man must validate his titles at the great intertribal feasts, the potlatches, where he is drawn into ever more strenuous commitments.

The institutions that arose in response to these values and goals are also similar in many respects. Loss of prestige and its symbols, rank and property, created such shame among the Kwakiutl and the Japanese that even the children responded by committing suicide. Murder as a means to goals or to avenge an insult was also institutionalized in the three societies.

Organized warfare was prevalent not because of lack of resources or for defensive purposes, but as an inevitable concomitant of group competitiveness and aggression. Cannibalism, human sacrifice and headhunting expressed the integration of religion and war among the Kwakiutl and the Ibo. Relations between the Kwakiutl and their gods also re-

---

[1]Sources of information about the Japanese were: Caudill (1959), Fletcher (1928), Haring (1948), Lemert (1962), Norbeck and De Vos (1961), Sikkema (1948).

[2]Sources of information about the Scots of the Hebrides Islands were: Beckwith (1962, 1969), MacLeish (1970), McPhee (1969), Morgenstern (1953).

flected the social tensions and were fraught with aggression and rivalry. Kwakiutl gods and Japanese Bushido manifested the cultural contempt for weakness. Bushido and ancestor worship made religious virtues of the feudal-militaristic values of obedience and loyalty to a superior among the Japanese, and Christianity reinforced the Ibo value of striving for success.

The values of the marketplace underlie the institution of marriage, for in all three societies women are objects of exchange. The increasing economic independence of Ibo women recently began to undermine their traditional legal, moral, and religious subordination, but the subordination of Japanese women is supported by industry and the professions. The Ibo and the Japanese woman can obtain a divorce only with great difficulty.

The family structure in the three societies is marked by tension and insecurity. Among the Ibo these are generated by the changing socioeconomic relations between husbands and wives. Among the Kwakiutl and Japanese the system of primogeniture causes bitter hatreds and rivalries, and the eldest Ibo son inherits not only his father's goods but also the debts, which may have accrued from his grandfather. The rivalry between Kwakiutl fathers and their daughters' husbands over the acquisition and repayment of titles often led to warfare between families and tribes. Tension prevails among the Japanese son, his mother and his wife, and the suppression of aggression in the hierarchical, patriarchal, Japanese family falls with the greatest force upon the women.

Kwakiutl children were inducted into the competitive potlatch pattern at an early age, and were hurried toward an aggressive, competing adulthood. The harsh physical punishment of these children for the violation of religious rules was exceptional among North American Indians. Young Ibo and Japanese children are greatly indulged, but school entrance creates a major discontinuity. School-age Japanese children become representatives of the family to the outside world. They must bring honor and glory to the family, never shame or ridicule. Ibo and Japanese children must achieve academically, for education is the key to their upward mobility. The Ibo boy assumes adult responsibilities at puberty, and must thenceforth make money at all costs to discharge religious, social, and economic obligations, to purchase titles, and to accumulate the bride-price. If a Kwakiutl or Japanese child failed to meet cultural demands, he might commit suicide.

Neither the Kwakiutl nor the Japanese tolerate abnormalities or imperfections. In the three societies, stuttering was an occupational and social liability even before contact with Europeans. The Kwakiutl and Ibo deride stuttering, and the Japanese are shamed by it. The Ibo and Kwakiutl place a very high premium on oratorical ability, and speech-making begins before adolescence. In Japan stuttering is part of a syndrome termed "anthrophobia" by Japanese psychiatrists, which expresses anxiety, inadequacy, and fear of meeting people.

The incidence of stuttering might constitute an "index of culture stress," said Naroll (1959:108), if there were sufficient data about stuttering. Culture stress is defined in terms of whether the culture is "tough" or "easy." This depends upon the number of paths to the goals of the culture and how difficult or easy it is for the individual to achieve these goals.

Psychological tension depends upon and varies with the properties of paths as means of reducing tension; and where a culture's paths make for easy tension-reduction in its members the culture is easy. Conversely where a culture's paths make for difficult tension-reduction the culture is tough (Arsenian and Arsenian [1948:379]).

It appears that the stuttering societies have cultures that are "tough." Stuttering seems to stem from the anxiety, fear, and frustration of the children in these societies as they attempt to achieve the personality and goals prescribed by their cultures.

CULTURAL PROFILE OF THE NONSTUTTERING SOCIETIES

The nonstuttering societies also share similar values, in contrast to the differences in their socioeconomic and ecological environments.

The aboriginal, Shoshonean-speaking Ute were a hunting and gathering people who lived principally in the Great Basin of North America, an area sparse in plant and animal life. With the advent of the horse and mounted buffalo hunting, their material culture expanded. But when the buffalo were exterminated, the Ute were forced onto reservations, where some still live in poverty-stricken migratory bands. The acculturated Ute are sedentary farmers, however, and many are prosperous leaders of their people.

The Hausa have for centuries been mainly farmers and traders, living in traditional, conservative, hierarchical chiefdoms, even under British rule.

The war-like, aggressive, Scottish clans were broken by the English in the middle of the eighteenth century. A short time later, when sheepherding became profitable, the surviving chiefs cleared many of the clansmen, their tenant farmers, out of the highlands and the islands. Not until a hundred years later did the remaining tenant farmers receive legal tenure to the land they worked. Now, however, that most people expect more from life than the bare necessities, farming no longer provides an adequate livelihood, and the immigration that began near the end of the eighteenth century has accelerated to such an extent that many of the Hebrides Islands have become depopulated. Those who remain on the islands are mainly farmers, fishermen, and shepherds, who receive welfare aid when they are in need.

The Ute, the Hausa, and the Scots are organized into highly cooperative societies, based on the extended family as the essential socioeconomic unit. Land ownership and the instruments of production are vital to the Hausa, but the Ute did not recognize territorial imperatives as they roamed the deserts and mountains in search of food, and most of the people in the Hebrides do not own the land they farm.

Internecine warfare between the Scottish clans came to an end more than two centuries ago, and neither the Ute nor the Hausa waged war for territorial aggrandizement, prestige, or honor. The Ute fought only defensively against more aggressive Indians, and the Hausa maintained their political sovereignty mainly by diplomatic means and the payment of tribute.

For the Ute and the Hausa, religion presents an orderly, coherent, and harmonious view of the cosmos, is completely integrated with social, political, and economic life, and offers institutionalized solutions for personal and group problems. Few of the Ute have converted to Christianity. The Hausa were converted to Islam in easy, uncoerced stages by their own religious teachers and integrated their pagan spirits with those of Islam. The Scots, who once worshipped the sun under the Celtic Druids, were in due course converted to Catholicism and then to Calvinism. Although the islanders are generally pious churchgoers, not many are now deeply religious. They easily shed Calvinist constraint, and lapse into blasphemy, hard drinking, bawdiness, and sexual freedom.

Ute men and women were equally engaged in the important economic activities and had about equal status. A type of "brittle monogamy" characterized most of their marriages; spouses were changed frequently, and divorce effected simply by a return to the parental camp.

Hausa marriage is polygynous, but although the women are legally minors and the wards of their husbands, they obtain a divorce as easily as the men. Muslim men may have no more than four wives at a time, but the women average three divorces in a lifetime. Hausa women use wife-seclusion to gain freedom from hard farm labor and leisure for handicrafts production, and retain the money they earn for their own use. They also violate wife-seclusion by intercompound visiting, and often leave the compound for long visits with their own kinfolk.

The Hebridean Scots are monogamous, but marriages frequently take place very shortly before the birth of the first child, and they are not stigmatized. Both the men and the women in the Hebrides do strenuous physical labor, and women of all ages pride themselves on their ability to carry heavy loads on their backs. At the parties which they hold as often as possible, the women encourage the men to drink so they will lose their sexual inhibitions; the women are acknowledged to be more highly sexed than the men.

In the three cultures the family is extended, the community is well integrated, and when a parent dies or is divorced the child is assured of surrogate parents. Children are loved and indulged. Ute parents accept their children's verbal aggression, and kin other than parents discipline the children by mild ridicule and threats of the supernatural. The Hausa and the Scottish boys are punished physically, the Hausa by the paternal uncle, and the Scots by parents and teachers. Hausa boys and girls of nine or ten go on remarkably free jaunts in the countryside, unsupervised by adults, entertain villagers by singing, and engage in incidental sexual play. Hausa girls also trade at an early age in the market, where they meet their suitors, and the wife-seclusion that follows marriage is, with all its compensations, sharply discontinuous. Out of the one-room schoolhouses and the small, crowded crofts in the Hebrides has come a disproportionate number of university honors scholars.

The Ute and the Hausa value adult oratorical ability, but their criterion for fluency is unhurried, deliberate, grave, thoughtful speech. Although the role of the Orator or Bard was once institutionalized in the Hebrides, speech fluency does not now help an individual to gain social or political prestige unless he has the requisite character and personality.

The three cultures accept their children as satisfactory speakers no matter how they speak and are very tolerant of linguistic variations. The Ute use a special diminutive, affectionate language with children, which encourages repetition. The Hausa believe that the listener has more of an obligation to understand what the speaker is saying than the speaker has to be intelligible. The Scots regard slowness of speech as an individual personality trait and are not concerned about the possibility that a child will stutter. Above all, the Ute, the Hausa, and the Scottish children are permitted freedom of speech and action. The Hausa speak their own language in primary school, but many of the Gaelic-speaking Scottish children learn English as a second language when they enter school.

In sum, the nonstuttering societies are cooperative. Prestige among the Ute and the Hausa depends on age and experience, and eventually comes to all. For men of special talent, leadership roles are available, but they are not achieved through competition and aggression. The Scots value cooperation as highly as competition, but the individual is independent and permitted to be idiosyncratic in behavior. The three cultures have institutionalized devices to relieve stress. None is time-oriented. All value generosity, hospitality, and sexual freedom. The Ute have their shamans, who support, heal, and sustain both the individual and the group. Hausa women compensate for their lack of freedom in a number of ways. And the Scots use gossip, parties, and alcohol as enjoyable outlets for their stresses.

Although the paths to social goals are no longer as clear and open as they once were because of the impact of social change, the non-stuttering societies are still "easy" cultures.

CHAPTER 4

Methodology, Procedures, and Statistical Findings

No island-wide survey of the incidence of stuttering in Puerto Rico had ever been made as of February, 1968, and at that time there were no special services for speech defects in the public schools. This is hardly surprising in view of the fact that the basic educational goal for the past three decades has been the elimination of illiteracy. In 1950 only half the school-age population was attending school, but by 1960, 91 percent of children aged six to twelve were enrolled in the public schools. For a number of years one-third of the Commonwealth budget has been spent on education, but the enormous strides made in basic education are still very recent.

Procedures in San Juan

To obtain the data on the incidence of stuttering in the public elementary schools of San Juan, I conducted a survey in person. I was authorized by the Regional Director of the San Juan Metropolitan School District to visit a sufficient number of schools to determine the incidence of stuttering in a population of 10,000 pupils in grades one through six. The Office of the Regional Director provided me with a list of schools representing a cross-section of the enrollment in the Metropolitan School District, and I obtained permission from the principals of these schools to determine the incidence of stuttering among their pupils. I sent these principals letters for the teachers in each school, explaining the purposes of the study and providing a definition of stuttering in both Spanish and English. I also sent them a questionnaire for the data on stuttering incidence in each class. To make certain that no child who stuttered would be overlooked, I asked the teachers to refer not only children who stuttered but also those who had any type of speech defect.

I found it necessary to visit a total of 12 schools in San Juan, with enrollments ranging from 533 to 1,792 children, to obtain the required population of 10,000. Each teacher in the 12 schools supplied the data on the number of children in her class who stuttered or had other speech defects, and the age and sex of each child. The school administrations furnished the data on enrollment, sex ratio, and a general statement about the socioeconomic level of the population, based on fathers' occupations. The socioeconomic level was very low, occasionally reaching the lower middle class as the top stratum.

I administered a speech screening test in Spanish and English to each child identified by the classroom teacher as having a speech defect. The test consisted of a series of questions designed to elicit responses which would include all the speech sounds in both languages. Each child also read, in front of the class, passages in Spanish and English from books he was currently using in school. In addition, I screened the speech of about 25 percent of the children in each school, selecting the classes at random. When I found a child who had a speech defect but had not been referred by his teacher, I tested the speech of each child in that class.

Procedures in New York City

Speech services for the New York City public schools were instituted in 1916 and are directed by the Bureau for Speech Improvement. Teachers of speech improvement diagnose and try to correct speech disorders, including stuttering. They hold either a bachelor's or master's degree in speech correction, and a substitute or regular license as teachers of speech improvement, based on examinations given by the Board of Examiners, Board of Education, City of New York.

The director of the Bureau for Speech Improvement authorized me to collect data on stuttering from the teachers of speech improvement in the New York City schools, and provided a list of these teachers.

The acting director of the Bureau of Educational Research authorized me to obtain data from school records pertaining to the length of residence of Puerto Rican children on the mainland. The Office of Integration and Human Relations provided a list of schools with an enrollment of at least 50 percent Puerto Rican children.

To obtain a population of 10,000 Puerto Rican children in grades one through six who had lived on the mainland for at least three years and were therefore somewhat acculturated, I obtained data on the length of mainland residence of the Puerto Rican children in each of 19 schools.

I sent letters to the speech improvement teachers in the 19 schools, explaining the study's purposes and requesting their cooperation. On a questionnaire which I provided, these teachers entered the data on stuttering incidence among the Puerto Rican children who had lived on the mainland for at least three years, as well as the grade, sex, and age of each child.

At the beginning or end of each school year, teachers of speech improvement routinely test the speech of all the children in the schools to which they are assigned. Their testing procedures and methods, standardized by the Bureau for Speech Improvement, are identical with those I used in the San Juan public schools.

Stuttering Incidence in San Juan

The incidence of stuttering among 10,449 children, consisting of 5,476 boys and 4,973 girls in grades one to six in the 12 public schools in the San Juan Metropolitan School District, was found to be 1.50 percent. The number of stutterers was 157: 119 boys and 38 girls. The incidence of stuttering in the male population was 2.17 percent; in the female population, 0.76 percent. The sex ratio was 2.9:1. Table 4.1 shows the number and sex of stutterers by grade.

Table 4.1—Stuttering Incidence in San Juan by Grade and Sex

Grade	Male	Female	Totals
1	22	4	26
2	17	6	23
3	16	7	23
4	28	10	38
5	17	6	23
6	19	5	24
	119	38	157

Stuttering Incidence in New York City

The incidence of stuttering among 10,455 Puerto Rican children, consisting of 5,270 boys and 5,185 girls, mainland residents for three years or more, in grades one to six in the 19 New York City schools, was 0.84 percent. The number of stutterers was 88: 76 boys and 12 girls.

The incidence of stuttering in the male population was 1.44 percent; in the female population, 0.23 percent. The sex ratio was 6.3:1. Table 4.2 shows the number and sex of stutterers by grade.

Table 4.2—Stuttering Incidence in New York by Grade and Sex

Grade	Male	Female	Totals
1	20	2	22
2	7	2	9
3	11	0	11
4	18	5	23
5	11	1	12
6	9	2	11
	76	12	88

Table 4.3—Summary of Data on Stuttering Incidence
in San Juan and New York

	San Juan	New York
Population	10,449	10,455
Boys	5,476	5,270
Girls	4,973	5,185
No. of Stutterers	157	88
Boys	119	76
Girls	38	12
Stuttering Incidence	1.50%	0.84%
Boys	2.17%	1.44%
Girls	0.76%	0.23%
Male-Female Ratio	2.9:1	6.3:1
San Juan-New York Male Ratio	1.5:1	
San Juan-New York Female Ratio	3.3:1	

Table 4.3 summarizes the data on stuttering incidence among Puerto Rican public elementary school children in San Juan and New York City.

The range of stuttering among school children in the United States is 0.6 percent to 1 percent (Johnson 1967), and the stuttering incidence among the Puerto Rican children in New York falls within this range. However, in San Juan stuttering incidence is about two and a half times that of the minimum and one and a half times that of the maximum in the United States. The stuttering incidence of Puerto Rican boys both in San Juan and New York exceeds the range in the United States. The stuttering incidence of the San Juan girls falls within this range, but for

Puerto Rican girls in New York stuttering incidence falls below the range.

Total stuttering incidence in San Juan was found to be almost twice that in New York. It was about one and a half times greater for San Juan boys than for the Puerto Rican boys in New York, but for the San Juan girls, 3.3 times greater than that of the Puerto Rican girls in New York. The difference between male and female stuttering in New York was found to be more than twice the difference in San Juan.

Also noteworthy is the fact that *both* in San Juan and New York City the highest stuttering incidence occurred in the fourth grade, and the next highest, in the first grade. The incidence of stuttering in the fourth grade in San Juan was considerably higher than in any of the other grades.

Statistical Significance of Differences in Stuttering Incidence

Using chi-square ($\times^2$) values (Underwood 1954), the differences in incidence of stuttering are clearly significant, as follows:

The difference in stuttering incidence between Puerto Rican children in grades one through six in the public schools in New York City and those in San Juan is significant at less than the 1 percent level of confidence ($\times^2 = 19.703$).

The difference in stuttering incidence between males in the New York population and males in the San Juan population is significant at less than the 1 percent level of confidence ($\times^2 = 8.054$).

The difference in stuttering incidence between females in the New York population and females in San Juan is significant at less than the 1 percent level of confidence ($\times^2 = 14.706$).

The difference in stuttering incidence between the total of males in New York City and San Juan and the total of females in New York City and San Juan is significant at less than the 1 percent level of confidence ($\times^2 = 78.839$).

The difference in stuttering incidence between males and females in the New York City population is significant at less than the 1 percent level of confidence ($\times^2 = 45.900$).

The difference in stuttering incidence between males and females in the San Juan population is significant at less than the 1 percent level of confidence ($\times^2 = 34.960$).

The difference between the male-female ratio in New York City and that in San Juan is significant at the 5 percent level of confidence ($\times^2 = 3.877$).

The Hypothesis and the Findings

I hypothesized that stuttering incidence would be higher among the Puerto Rican children in New York City than in San Juan on the assumption that the acculturation of the rural migrants in New York would be more stressful than their urbanization in San Juan. Surveys in San Juan and New York, however, revealed a higher incidence of stuttering in San Juan, statistically significant below the 1 percent level of confidence. When I examined and compared the two milieus to discover the sociocultural and economic variables and stresses, I found that I had not sufficiently taken into account the importance of the differences in the dominant values of Puerto Rico and the United States, as well as the benefits to the migrants of acculturation in New York.

In investigating indicators of cultural stress, Naroll (1959:108) found that "data on four categories proved rich enough for use": suicide, homicide, alcoholism, and witchcraft. "Five other categories proved disappointing; there were not enough data in the files" on narcotics addiction, personality disorders, offenses against the mores other than homicide, psychosomatic illnesses, and stuttering. The statistically significant differences in stuttering incidence among Puerto Rican elementary school children in San Juan and New York City, as found in this study, may be considered an index to differences in sociocultural and economic stress for Puerto Rican migrants in San Juan and New York.

PART II

PUERTO RICO:
CULTURAL-HISTORICAL PERSPECTIVE

CHAPTER 5

The Spanish Heritage and the North American Overlay

Puerto Ricans migrate to San Juan and New York City from the highlands and coasts of Puerto Rico, and their cultural patterns and values, modified by urban life, underlie the stresses which create stuttering among their children. These values evolved in the Iberian region of Europe several thousand years ago. They were altered by the Latin American experience, and gradually took on a peculiarly Puerto Rican cast in the context of the island's history. They were again changed by the coming of the Americans.

The Spanish Heritage

The colonizers of both Puerto Rico and the United States came from the same culture area, Europe, and all Europeans shared the same religion, Catholicism, well into the sixteenth century. Even during the Moorish occupation Spain remained part of the circum-Mediterranean culture, and Spanish cities, architecture, culture, and folklore reflect European forms. Above all, the basic family pattern in Spain is European: "Spain is Europe and Spaniards are European" (Foster 1960:29).

In Spain, Catholicism exercised a more profound influence than in the other Catholic countries. Peninsular industrialization proceeded at a much slower pace than in northern Protestant Europe during the four centuries in which Spain shaped the sociocultural and economic configurations of its colonies in the America.

Until the nineteenth century, Spain barricaded its empire from contact with the rest of the world in order to maintain its monopoly over trade with its colonies. And when Puerto Rico was found to have few mineral resources, the island became even more isolated than the other Spanish colonies. Puerto Rico came to be used principally as a garrison post and supply depot, and only its widespread smuggling operations with the other Caribbean islands provided contact with the outside world.

Exclusion from foreign trade and commerce . . . involved exclusion from foreign cultural and intellectual influence. Similarly, denial of commercial reciprocity between homeland and colony drew in its wake denial of intellectual and cultural reciprocity (G. Lewis 1963:53–54).

Not only was Puerto Rico denied a university, but its youth was strongly discouraged from attending schools anywhere but in Spain to prevent contact with non-Spanish contemporary thought. And non-Catholics were not permitted to immigate into the island.

The earliest settlers in Puerto Rico were mainly discredited soldiers and priests. "Madrid used overseas appointments to rid itself of socially disgraced or politically undesirable individuals" (G. Lewis 1963:52). Gradually the population was increased by deserting sailors, stowaways, former prisoners, slaves fleeing from the other Antilles islands, royalists escaping from the revolutions in South America, and Catholic entrepreneurs from the United States and Middle and South America.

When the Spanish came to Puerto Rico at the beginning of the sixteenth century, they found an egalitarian agricultural society of Arawak Indians, whom they promptly enslaved for work in the mines and fields, even though officially the Church opposed slavery. Some of the Indians managed to escape to the mountains, but the native population soon declined because of the enforced hard labor, unsuccessful resistance to the Spanish, and exposure to European diseases. By the beginning of the eighteenth century, the remaining Arawak had been culturally and physically assimilated and disappeared as a distinct racial stock. Throughout this period Spanish men and Indian women intermingled, leaving a heritage which still persists in the physical features, speech, and probably some of the religious practices of present-day Puerto Ricans.

With the introduction of chocolate from the New World and the increasing popularity of coffee in Europe, sugar had become the most valuable agricultural commodity in international trade, and the Spanish soon discovered that the lowlands and coastal plains of the island could be used to grow sugarcane. Since the decrease of the native population resulted in a labor shortage, several thousand slaves were brought in from Africa early in the sixteenth century. To circumvent the religious sanctions against direct slave trading, the Crown issued licenses to trading companies, which bought slaves from other Europeans.

Catholic leaders in Puerto Rico, however, did not actively sanction a chattel status for the black; they neither segregated him, nor made a religious issue out of his race. White males outnumbered white females by two to one during the first century of the colonial period, and "from the beginning the Spanish settlers had had no prejudice against intermarriage with either Indians or mulattoes. The mixed society thus created, although scornful of Negro, at the same time became more and more tolerant of the social advance of the colored man with talent" (G. Lewis 1963:58). Upper-class fathers sometimes educated their colored offspring and left them property. During the eighteenth century, equal public education was legally established for mulatto and white children (Williams 1945:308–317). Thus it came about that "the free colored class . . . preferred to seek the approbation of their white superiors rather than risk social opprobrium by identifying themselves with the Negro population" (G. Lewis 1963:61).

Since the island was used primarily as a military outpost, plantation agriculture was not permitted to develop nearly as extensively as in the other Caribbean islands, and the number of slaves who were imported never exceeded the number who were freed. With most of the land in the royal domain, slaves who were freed by their masters or who performed military service, because squatter farmers, or *agregados,* resident workers, on a plantation. Interracial mixing prevailed throughout the lower class, which did not stigmatize either the consensual unions between blacks and whites, or their offspring.

By the beginning of the nineteenth century, when commercial agriculture and cattle raising had developed more fully, the slave population had tripled. But by this time the number of free blacks was also large not only because of manumission but also because Puerto Rico had for long been a refuge for slaves escaping from neighboring islands, who were given small tracts of land if they accepted Catholicism. About the middle of the nineteenth century, when the number of slaves reached a peak, there were three and a half times as many free blacks in Puerto Rico as slaves. Nominally free workers, however, both black and white, were reduced to a virtual slave status by labor laws that bound them to the soil as *peons.* Thus, so-called free workers, both black and white, performed the same labor side by side with slaves.

With an adequate supply of "free" labor and the introduction of labor-saving devices, slave labor became uneconomical on the plantations. Thus the owners of the larger sugar plantations supported the abolition of slavery, which became part of the movement for political autonomy. "The integration of Negro subgroups into Puerto Rican nationality thus came to be closely tied to the fight for greater self-determination on the part of the Island" (Steward 1956:497).

Although all races were guaranteed legal and political equality when slavery was abolished in 1873, mulattoes had much greater social and economic mobility than blacks. Moreover, socioeconomic class was decisive. A wealthy or politically prominent mulatto was socially defined as white, but a poor mulatto was labeled black. Nevertheless "conditions for the integration of the Negro after emancipation were more favorable in Puerto Rico than in any other Caribbean territory except the Dominican Republic" (Mintz 1956:410). Negro slaves had received better technical training than the white *agregados* and day laborers, and after slavery was abolished, blacks continued to work as artisans:

their importance in supplying the needed skills for insular industrial development lingers on in the common belief that Negroes are innately more clever than whites or are endowed with greater mechanical aptitude (Williams 1945:309).

For four centuries the Catholic Church played a very important role in molding the social institutions in Puerto Rico.

San Juan, on the urgent request of its very first bishop, had been the first bishopric in the New World to receive into its hands the authority of the Catholic Inquisition (G. Lewis 1963:60).

But the Spanish Crown played off the colonial army against the Church. Although the army was paid by the king, the Church had to support itself. But since the population in Puerto Rico was dispersed and roads were few and poor, the Church could collect few tithes easily, and the clergy derived part of their income from buying and selling both Indian and black slaves.

Despite the power of the Church, religious orthodoxy was weak in Puerto Rico from the beginning. A number of upper-class, anti-Spanish Puerto Ricans were drawn to the rationalist movements of eighteenth-century Europe, and still others were Spiritualists. The lower classes, conspicuously isolated from the dominant groups, retained the medieval Spanish cult of the Virgin and the saints, mixed with Indian and Negro beliefs in magic, and the majority attended church only for a christening, a wedding or a funeral. Many rural workers, anti-Spanish because they were exploited by the Spanish landowners, also became anti-Catholic when the Church helped to implement the repressive labor laws. These workers secretly practiced Protestantism, which had been brought into Puerto Rico by the few English settlers.

In the middle of the nineteenth century, Church property was expropriated and Catholic influence was further weakened. When the local clergy in a number of Latin American countries participated in the anti-Spanish revolutions, the Puerto Rican government began to import priests from Spain. The Spanish priests regarded administering the sacraments their basic function, and traditionally remained aloof from the problems of the poor. "By 1898, certainly, the gulf between the populace and Church was complete" (G. Lewis 1963).

By this time the landless population of the island was very large. With only 21 percent of the land under cultivation, more than 35 percent of the cultivated land was owned by .025 percent of the landowners, and 10 percent, by 56 percent of the farmers (Steward 1956:57). The large landowners, who grew coffee in the highlands and raised sugarcane and cattle on the coast, determined the rural social structure. Also in the upper class were the military, the priesthood, administrative officials, and a group of powerful merchants who supplied the landowners with credit. All were generally white, Catholic, and Spanish or Spanish-oriented.

The lowest socioeconomic group, the largest class by far, consisted of the small independent farmers, the *agregados,* and the rural and urban wage laborers. Although the number of small farmers had decreased, they were still numerous in the many parts of the island which could not be used for *hacienda* agriculture. Many of these farmers had also begun to grow cash crops, such as tobacco, so that they could buy the manufactured goods which were being imported in increasing quantities.

The lower classes constituted "a unique pre-industrial . . . peasant class so typical of Puerto Rican society even today," as Gordon Lewis expresses it. From their early ancestors the masses had inherited "an anti-social individualism" and were interested only in their own "personal protection and personal advancement." Under Spanish colonialism they were morally passive, for the island had not been permitted to develop in any way that would benefit the majority of the people. After four centuries of Spanish rule, Puerto Rico had neither banks nor effective circulation of money, only two or three roads and a small strip of railroad track.

Without schools, without books whose importation is banned by the Customs, without metropolitan newspapers whose circulation is suppressed, without political representation, without municipal self-government, lacking either thought or conscience, the physical and mental energies of our people are exclusively absorbed in the production of sugar to sell to England and the United States; Puerto Rico is simply a factory openly exploited (G. Lewis 1963:61).

But the growing middle class—the doctors, lawyers, teachers, and journalists—"contributed . . . extensively to the intellectual life of the capital and to the liberal-reformist movement" (G. Lewis 1963:56–61). As agriculture, commerce, and government expanded, a number of towns came into being, and as regional crop specialization intensified, a town-country pattern evolved and new values emerged.

Increasingly, personal wealth became the goal, and the individual felt personally responsible for his success or failure. These attitudes were reflected in new standards of living, new forms of interpersonal relations, and even in the adoption of a new ... value orientation ... the Protestant ethic (Steward 1956:60–61).

Nevertheless, certain aspects of the Spanish heritage persisted relatively unchanged even after the American occupation. These aspects, which transcended class lines, were the language, the importance of the extended family, ritual kinship, male dominance, and the double sex standard.

The Latin American Ethos

In the face of cultural and historical events that were essentially similar throughout Latin America, some facets of the Spanish heritage were minimized, some were exaggerated, and some were transformed. Thus there emerged a Latin American ethos, shared by Puerto Rico, with emphases that differed from those of the original model.

The Spanish, like other Catholics, believe that every individual has a soul and therefore has intrinsic worth. The New World conqueror, a marginal man without ascribed status, exaggerated the value of individuality as he emphasized his own individual worth. This view was syncretized with the American Indian concept of the soul as guardian spirit, and accounted for the supreme importance of individuality in Latin America.

The essence of the individual, his soul, is expressed by the value of *dignidad,* which is guarded from insult and invasion by *respeto,* a pattern of ceremonial politeness constantly observed by all but the closest relatives and friends. "Personal and national pride are great, and dignity and face must be preserved at all costs" (Foster 1960:4). In their relationships with social inferiors, those in the upper strata usually honor the creed of *dignidad* and *respeto:*

almost all persons in superordinate positions, whose statuses involve human relations and who expect to hold them longer than momentarily on any other basis than naked force, do follow the culture pattern of at least ostensibly respecting the inner uniqueness of others, even subordinates (Gillin 1955:491).

Although social inequality and class stratification are accepted, everyone has "the obligation to ... try to realize the aspirations his inner integrity demands" (Gillin 1955:491). In all classes the *macho* is the ideal personality for which men strive. The *macho* is the man who is confident of his inner worth and who expresses this confidence in action or, if he is an intellectual or a politician, in words. The complete *macho* may become a *caudillo* because he personifies the aspirations of other men. Freedom of action and the emphasis on individualism are sometimes carried to such great lengths by Latin American men that they approach anarchy.

Important interpersonal relationships are categorized in terms of the reciprocal obligations involved. Kinship, both consanguine and affinal, is the primary bond, and prescribes the strongest rights and duties. Mutual responsibilities between godparents and godchildren, and between godparents and parents, are sanctified by *compadrazgo,* a religious institution, and *compadres* enjoy joking privileges that are not permitted in more formal relationships. *Confianza* expresses pure friendship, based on mutual understanding and appreciation, without the obligations of kinship, either real or fictive.

Impersonal relationships between human beings are anathema to Latin Americans, who prefer to relate to the larger society through *personalismo,* the connections radiating out from the personal relationships with relatives and friends. "At one and the same time," says Gillin (1955:497), ". . . the average Latin American is motivated to maintain the established order and also to take advantage of it for his own personal ends with the help of his friends, including kinsmen."

The Latin American regards work as a necessary evil, which must be done in order to live, but which is to be avoided if one is wealthy or lucky. Verbal proficiency and manipulation are much more highly admired than scientific and technical ability, and the philosopher and poet have higher status than the scientist and engineer. "The Word is more valued than the Thing in modern Latin American culture" (Gillin 1955:499).

So-called typical Latin American values and behavior, nevertheless, characterize the upper classes and not the majority of the people. Only the upper classes have enough wealth to disdain manual labor, enough education to value the humanities, and enough connections to achieve power and other benefits.

The less affluent and less privileged groups never had to decide whether to shun manual labor in favor of upper-class occupations. They never had the chance to cultivate poetry and philosophy, for they were illiterate. . . . They did not face the issue of whether to be materialistic, for the only life they knew was one of daily toil (Steward 1956:491).

Although the upper strata may respect the *dignidad* of their social inferiors, the subordinate, dependent position of the lower class in the traditional two-class system of Latin America is reflected in every institution—in the relations between the state and the people, the Church and the people, employers and employees, husbands and wives, parents and children.

The parent-child relationship, in which the authority of age and life-long obedience to that authority were the main principles, was the keystone of the whole relational system. And, as is so often the case where these principles are found, there was a clear-cut dominance of the male over the female (F. Kluckhohn and Strodtbeck 1961:196).

The North American Overlay

The American occupation accelerated trends that were already under way in Puerto Rico, and initiated new ones.

These changes were imposed from above and from the outside by carriers of another culture, sometimes ruthlessly, sometimes disruptively, and in all cases in a way requiring quick adaptation (Steward 1956:79).

All aspects of Puerto Rican life were affected. Trade and industry expanded, government services increased, new towns appeared, education spurted, and the middle class grew. New medical and welfare services were introduced; the death rate dropped and the birth rate soared. But the most important result of economic and political dependency on the United States was the decreased self-sufficiency of Puerto Rico and its more efficient and intensive development as an agrarian economy. By 1930 economic concentration and absentee ownership were highly developed.

In the field of public utilities and banking the degree of absentee ownership by American corporations was some 60%; in the tobacco industry, 80%; in the sugar industry, 60%; and in the steamship lines operating between the island ports and the mainland ports, almost 100% (G. Lewis 1963:94).

The mainland-owned companies took enormous wealth from the island in dividends and profits and paid very low taxes to the insular government. The most lucrative jobs went to the continentals, not to the Puerto Ricans. The masses of agricultural workers were forced into seasonal work for American corporations and were deprived of the paternalism that protected them "from the worst of the onslaughts of rural life." Although the federal government had spent about $50 million in the island by 1930, it "concentrated most heavily upon appropriations for public works projects . . . and therefore did little more than touch the surface of the deeper social and economic ills." In 1935, Secretary Harold Ickes wrote: "There is today more widespread misery and destitution and far more unemployment in Puerto Rico than at any previous time in its history" (G. Lewis 1963:92–98).

Although race prejudice antedated the American occupation, the influx of American capital into Puerto Rico exacerbated discrimination, especially in higher-paid private employment. By 1943 discrimination had increased to such an extent that the legislature passed a Civil Rights Act.

Service in the American army during World War II brought Puerto Ricans into direct contact with American racial and ethnic prejudice. White Puerto Ricans objected to being classified with dark-skinned Puerto Ricans because this relegated them to an inferior status. Black Puerto Ricans "were subjected to the additional humiliation and indignities of segregation suffered by virtually all Negro troops in the American army" (Manners 1956:258). Most Puerto Ricans had to serve under American officers, whom they disliked violently. In spite of the benefits they received, veterans were united by their resentment against Americans into the groups working actively for Puerto Rican independence.

Despite the fact that color is not openly denigrated, most dark-skinned Puerto Ricans, under both the Spanish and the Americans, have suffered from a "virulent sense of racial shame, disguising itself under a spurious and comic invocation of things Spanish" (G. Lewis 1963:284). They seek refuge in the claim that they are Indian, Spanish, or Latin, and ignore those among them who proclaim their race openly and with pride.

The superior social status of white Puerto Ricans is not necessarily recognized by Americans.

As American forms of discrimination press upon these more ambivalent forms, the Puerto Rican who regards himself as white will increasingly find himself in the cruelly ironic position of being himself subjected to the prejudicial techniques he has hitherto utilized against the dark-colored persons of his own society (G. Lewis 1963:284).

Civil liberties investigations in 1958–59 and in 1963 disclosed an increase of racial discrimination in some private schools, in college fraternities and sororities, in the more expensive housing developments, in the high-priced tourist hotels, and in banks. In sponsoring the 1958–59 inquiry, the commonwealth government was among the first in the world "to have sponsored voluntarily an independent investigation into its own domestic record, in this case under the auspices of the General Assembly of the United Nations" (G. Lewis 1963:348).

When the Americans occupied Puerto Rico, the Catholic Church was separated from the state and developed ties with American Catholicism. A number of middle-class civil servants, professionals and small merchants in the towns converted to Protestantism, but its "American middle-class morality" had little appeal for the rural and urban poor, who joined the revivalist sects in increasing numbers. The pastor in these sects is a lay leader who comes from the same class as his congregation and can be approached without the deference and etiquette due a Catholic priest. The members read the Bible together in Spanish and experience a sense of community and direct religious involvement. Like the early Protestant churches, the revivalist sects help to integrate their members into the developing capitalist society.

The various tenets and taboos add up not only to forced economic saving, but also to the idealization of deferred gratification . . . conversion may be viewed as a way of increasing one's social and economic mobility (Mintz 1960:266).

Although Spiritualism is condemned by the Catholic Church, it became increasingly popular in Puerto Rico. Its adherents, generally nominal Catholics whose traditional way of life has been disrupted by social change, include small farmers, rural and urban workers, and women schoolteachers who have risen from a lower economic class.

Since 1900 the population of Puerto Rico has almost trebled and now numbers about three million. Even with the vast migration to the mainland, where well over a million Puerto Ricans are living, population density is extremely high: 766 people per square mile, compared with 65 people per square mile on the mainland. Thus migration has been a safety valve of great importance for the island.

But since the middle 1960s, migration has slowed down and in some years is exceeded by an outflow back to Puerto Rico, primarily because of increasingly difficult economic conditions for Puerto Ricans on the mainland. Automation wiped out many of the unskilled and semiskilled jobs that were usually taken by the migrants, and the upgrading of educational requirements, training and language ability has left many first-generation Puerto Rican migrants behind.

Return migration probably aggravates the chronic unemployment in Puerto Rico, which oscillates between 8.3 percent and 15.6 percent (G. Lewis 1963:230) and is almost as severe as mainland unemployment during the depression of the 1930s. Those who return to the island because they are not able to earn a living in the United States experience the same difficulties in Puerto Rico, for mechanization has reduced employment opportunities in agriculture and on the docks faster than new industrial jobs have been created. "The establishment of industry in Puerto Rico cannot be based on labor-intensive plans if industry using primarily human labor in production fails to compete favorably with mechanized and automated industry" (Hernández-Alvarez 1967:8).

CHAPTER 6

Rural Subcultures in Puerto Rico

The Puerto Ricans migrate to San Juan and New York mainly from five representative subcultures: the coffee-growing western highlands, the tobacco and mixed-crops regions in the eastern highlands, privately owned sugar *haciendas,* the cooperative government-owned sugarcane farms on the north coast, and the corporation-owned sugarcane farms on the south coast. Although these subcultures share many of the common cultural denominators of the island, the cultural-ecological processes peculiar to each subculture produce variant values and stresses. These differing patterns are variously affected by the urban experience, are associated with varying types of stress, and differently affect stuttering incidence among the children.

The rural subcultures and the subcultures of the migrants in the urban areas together constitute what Redfield (1941) calls a modified "folk-urban continuum." In the 1940s and 1950s, when the migrants were themselves children, sugar and coffee *hacienda* agriculture, typified by the traditional landlord-peasant economy, represented one pole of the continuum. The coffee region particularly was marked by "isolation; a high degree of genetic and cultural homogeneity; slow culture change; . . . social organization based on blood and fictive kinship; behavior which is traditional and uncritical; . . . the pervasive importance of magic and religion" (Mintz 1953–54:137).

The medium and small tobacco farmers and sharecroppers were more affected by the values of a cash nexus than the traditional *hacienda,* and had more opportunity for upward mobility than the small farmers, *agregados,* and wage laborers in the other subcultures. The agricultural sugar workers on the privately owned *haciendas* and on the coast could achieve upward mobility only through migration. The coastal workers share many of the characteristics of the landless, propertyless, wage-earning, urban proletariat, and in some respects are the best prepared for their life in San Juan and New York City, the urban pole of the folk-urban continuum.

Common Cultural Denominators

Until the nineteenth century, the highlands were the open frontier of Puerto Rico. Here the squatter farmer—Indian, white, and black—lived on his subsistence crops, independent and isolated from the other social classes. When private property was instituted about the middle of the eighteenth century and sugarcane became an important commercial crop, the small farmer, the *jíbaro,* was pushed off the land on the coast, and could work on the new sugar plantations or move farther inland. When the coffee industry was established in the mountains, the *jíbaro* grew coffee on a small scale, but if he lost his property to the Spanish *hacendado,* he was forced to work on the *hacienda* or to migrate. As tobacco became an important cash crop, with the coming of the Americans, the sharecropper could sometimes acquire a little land, but the wage laborer had few such opportunities.

The production of sugar, coffee, and tobacco is marked by the *tiempo muerto,* and it is in the "dead time" after the crops are harvested that the *jíbaro* migrates, either temporarily or permanently. Throughout the agricultural areas subsidiary economic activities become particularly important during the *tiempo muerto,* and include raising livestock, mainly by women and children; needlework, by women and girls; making and selling illegal rum; and all forms of gambling, especially on the illegal lottery.

Under Spain, the small farmer lived in "moral and social degradation . . . as a forgotten and submerged person." Under the Americans his house remained dismal and ugly, and he was still disease ridden and undernourished. But the groups who profited from the *jíbaro* rationalized their expoitation of him.

Since he was natively shrewd, the town merchant was morally free to try to deceive him. Since he was said to be lazy when working for others, means to make him work had to be found. . . . Since he was so well acquainted with nature's remedies and he was supposed to be inherently healthy, he presumably did not require medical services. Since he was natively intelligent and resourceful, educational facilities were said to be wasted on him. And since he is a child of nature, rural roads, modern housing, schools, radios, high wages, and too much governmental service were said to ruin him. Civilization tempts him to leave the land. . . . As a consequence he . . . became a social liability as an urban slum dweller (Steward 1956:498).

Since 1940 the *jíbaro* has been the symbol of the Popular Democratic Party, which did much to improve the life of the rural population from which it drew a great deal of its strength. Nevertheless, the term *jíbaro* is derogatory and is used as a label for those who are regarded as backward and unsophisticated. The sugar workers on the coast are insulted when the townspeople refer to them as *jíbaros,* but the sugar workers apply the term to those who migrate to the coast from the highlands., It has come to include the small farmers and the many landless agricultural workers and sharecroppers who are the least educated and poorest of all the people in Puerto Rico. *Jíbaros* share certain cultural patterns regardless of crop specialization, as well as many of the common denominators of Puerto Rican culture.

The relationship between the *hacendado* and the *agregado* is rooted in *respeto.* The ideal landowner provides "life for the people" (Manners 1956:136). He furnishes the subsistence plot, a house, and work for the entire year. The *agregado* may obtain his supplies on credit if there is a store on the *hacienda,* and then becomes bound to the landowner by his indebtedness. The *hacendado* helps his workers in legal, medical, and political matters, may tell them how to vote, and sometimes becomes a *compadre* to their children.

The ideal worker is trustworthy, hardworking and competent. He must work whenever the landowner requires it, and must also put his family at the *hacendado*'s service without any necessary compensation. Frequently his wife works in the *hacienda* kitchen; his son runs errands for all members of the landowner's family; less frequently now than formerly, his daughter is called upon to donate her sexual services.

In 1898 about 92 percent of Puerto Rican children between the ages of five and 17 were illiterate. In the last year of the Spanish regime, the total amount of money spent on public education (about $20,000) was just equal to the salary of the Spanish governor according to Gordon Lewis (1963:55). Since 1900, from a quarter to a third of the insular budget has been spent on education. But the American form of education was imposed without regard for the special needs of the *jíbaro*'s children:

neither curriculum nor organizational structure . . . made any distinction between the education of the rural child and that of the urban child, with the consequence . . . that the former was sacrificed to the latter (G. Lewis 1963:442).

It was not until 1928 that the junior high school was established in the rural communities, and "as late as 1940" there was not a single senior high school in any of the 45 rural municipalities that contained some two-fifths of the total insular population. In addition, when the Commissioner of Education was an American, the bilingual emphasis resulted in educational chaos and ignorance of both Spanish and English.

Both rural and urban working-class children attend college and university in decreasing proportions as compared with previous years, and also as compared with middle- and upper-class children. "There is, even more, an increasing discrimination against the rural school child in favor of his urban and suburban counterpart" (G. Lewis 1963:463). In 1960, 64.8 percent of Puerto Ricans under the age of 25 had less than five years of schooling, compared with the average of 11 percent on the mainland (G. Lewis 1963:446). In the rural areas, 68.2 percent of the population had no more than four years of school and 2.3 percent went on to higher education, compared with 43.5 percent with no more than four years of school and 10.7 percent in higher education in the cities. And "rural-born, rural-resident persons have the least opportunity of obtaining a high-school education" (Tumin and Feldman 1961:43, 57).

The *jíbaro* respects learning and acknowledges the importance of literacy. But, in addition to the inadequate rural education, rural children are often taken out of school because they are needed for work in the fields or the house; because of illness, bad weather, lack of proper clothing; because a son must bring lunch to his father in the fields; or because the family migrates to another area in search of work. Also, since the parents themselves have little education, they stress proper behavior, not academic achievement, and are disappointed when learning does not take place automatically with school attendance. Moreover, they have no reason to believe that a little more education will make much difference in the future of their children.

Nevertheless, throughout Puerto Rico even a few years of education transmit the values of the changing society.

An "American" education instills standards of diet, behavior, material goods, conspicuous consumption, etiquette, social mobility, individual effort . . . which conform most closely to the behavior system of the middle and upper classes in town (Wolf 1956:254).

Most teachers are members of the lower middle or middle class, and as they "rise from the lower-stratum families, they tend to reveal intense hostility to lower-level habits" (G. Lewis 1963:448). Children of rural workers sometimes drop out of junior or senior high school in the towns because they are made to feel ashamed of their clothes, their speech, and their manners. But to many rural girls the role of the teacher is an attractive alternative to that of housewife on a farm.

The commonwealth government has established public health centers throughout the island, but provisions for the care of the aged are limited and the average older Puerto Rican is likely to be "a sickly and complaining person." He has "chronic ailments, long unattended," and "he is puzzled and bewildered by rapid social changes which gradually rob him of the status of the venerable patriarch afforded him by the older cultural milieu" (G. Lewis 1963:226).

There are few facilities for the mentally ill or deficient, who must generally stay with their families, and there is little education in preventive medicine. Despite a chronic shortage of doctors and nurses, the local medical association has opposed the efforts of the Secretary of Health to bring non-American doctors into the island, although Puerto Rican physicians migrate to the mainland in large numbers. Also, trained nurses much prefer to live in the towns than the rural areas. This leaves two-thirds of the island population medically indigent.

Even the rural doctors very rarely visit the isolated areas and, in any case, do not pay home visits to the poor. The more isolated folk in the highlands cannot easily get to the medical and health services in the rural towns, and when rural lower-class people do attend clinics, the nature of an illness or even the cause of a death is not discussed with them because they are considered too ignorant to understand. Since they anticipate a lack of respect and personal attention, many rural residents are reluctant to stay in a hospital. Thus folk theories about disease and folk remedies are perpetuated.

In addition to the inadequate care for the aged and the mentally ill, the shortage of doctors, dentists, and nurses in the rural areas, the lack of education in preventive medicine, the cavalier treatment of the rural poor, and the persistence of folk medicine, the health problems of rural people stem mainly from malnutrition and undernourishment, the consequences of poverty. The low protein value of the standard mixture of rice and beans accounts for the fact that the percentage of children suffering from intestinal parasites is substantially the same today as it was 40 years ago.

Throughout the rural areas, the cult of the Virgin and the saints is widespread. The saints are regarded as the intermediaries between man and God, who intercede for favors in exchange for pledges and acts of devotion. Spiritualism is also very popular, and the services of the Spiritualist medium have for the most part supplanted those of the traditional curer. The revivalist sects, especially the Pentecostals, are increasingly a source of moral, religious, and social support.

The Puerto Rican ambivalence toward race also prevails in the rural areas, where the ideal is light skin color, and no one wants to be identified as black or so identifies himself. Thus blacks suffer discrimination in upper-class employment, although they have equal opportunity in middle and lower-class jobs.

Compadrazgo has been secularized in many of the rural areas as the values of the cash economy replace unpaid ritual obligations, and sometimes the child is altogether omitted from the relationship. As agriculture declines in importance and the relationships between *hacendado* and *agregado* become more impersonal, ritual kinship is increasingly an intraclass bond among rural workers, or a tie between friends and family members. Even the secular bond is becoming attenuated with the greater emphasis on individual effort and cash payment for services.

The extended family is still important in all classes and regions, and for the rural and urban working class it constitutes an essential source of aid and services, especially in emergencies. However, like ritual kinship, even extended family bonds have weakened among those who have accepted individual competition as a primary value.

The Puerto Rican family, rooted in Spanish Catholicism, is imbued with "a male authoritarian ideal in which the husband has played the role of unquestioned *paterfamilias,* and the wife, especially at the proletarian levels, has had almost a chattel status." The twin sexual ideals of virginity for women and *machismo* for men have operated to maintain a rigid barrier between the sexes, preventing communication in many vital areas. The woman generally comes to marriage with fear concerning men and sex. The man expects his wife to be a mother substitute, for under the cover of *machismo* he retains his infantile dependence upon women. The puritanical attitude toward women, especially among lower-income groups, is coupled with intense male jealousy, for the obsession about female purity is accompanied by the conviction that a woman yields easily to sexual temptation. "The consequent strain frequently becomes unbearable, as indeed the high rate of suicide at this social level appears to bear out" (G. Lewis 1963:264–266).

In view of the tremendous importance placed on premarital chastity, the relatively high rate of consensual unions among lower-class Puerto Ricans appears paradoxical. But they do not see a religious or civil ceremony as relevant to the immediate problems of their lives, and common-law marriage is theoretically as binding as religious or civil marriage upon the birth of the first child. Nevertheless, even lower-class parents prefer their daughters to marry legally for greater prestige and economic protection. And when land ownership is connected with marriage, or when upward mobility is possible, or young men have fairly secure incomes, the legal ceremony is generally chosen.

Usually men are far more authoritarian in the highlands, where religious and civil marriage is customary, than on the coast, where common-law marriage is more frequent. Although every attempt is made to safeguard the chastity of girls and women, even in the highlands consensual unions increase as small farmers lose their land and swell the ranks of the agricultural workers. Thus common-law marriages occur most frequently where poverty is greatest. While many are permanent, they tend to be brittle, and when they are dissolved the children remain with the mother, frequently in a three-generation matrifocal household.

The popular assumptions about the causes of the high fertility rate in Puerto Rico were examined in a recent study and rejected as false. It is assumed:

(1) that Puerto Ricans have the large family values of an agricultural people; (2) that Puerto Rican males, especially, are obsessed with the desire to prove their masculinity by having many children . . . ; (3) that the lower classes are largely ignorant of birth control methods; and (4) that the influence of the Roman Catholic Church makes them not ready to utilize modern mechanical-chemical methods of family limitation (Hill, Stycos and Back 1959:328).

However, the ideal of the small family was found to be widespread, particularly among men. "In Puerto Rico, men are authoritarian, dominant, and distant, but not virility obsessed" (Hill et al. 1959:375).

The necessity for birth control was also generally accepted, and the insular health department had provided 160 public health units throughout Puerto Rico, "for its size . . . one of the most extensive systems of birth control in the world" (Hill et al. 1959:367). But it served less than 5 percent of the population, because the existence and location of the clinics, especially in the rural areas, were not publicized and because the personnel were neutral about the use of contraceptives.

Although staffed by Puerto Ricans, the clinics violated a number of cultural norms. The personnel discussed family planning only with the wives, threatening male dominance in the traditionally male-centered sexual sphere. Male physicians examined the women, violating their modesty, as well as offending the "protective, possessive, jealous" husbands (Hill et al. 1959:373). Above all, the clinic staffs ignored the respect barriers between husband and wife and their lack of communication on sexual matters. Further, the clinics frequently distributed defective contraceptives, did not stock a sufficient diversity or number, and enforced clinic hours too rigidly. Thus, after they already had large families, women were driven to sterilization, the contraceptive method most opposed by the Catholic Church.

Certain child-rearing patterns are widespread throughout the Puerto Rican rural lower classes. Babies are treated affectionately and indulgently. They are fed on demand and are generally not weaned until the next pregnancy. Children have few bedtime restrictions, and they participate in religious and family festivals even when they last all night. Children become physically independent and learn manual skills at an early age, and by the time they are five or six they go on errands alone.

They become aware of parental sexual relations when they are very young because of the lack of privacy in the small, crowded, rural huts. At the same time, sex differentiation in modesty training is begun very early. Baby girls are always covered, for males are viewed as sexually irresponsible, and incest is greatly feared.

there is an extremely close relationship in Puerto Rico between crime, mental illness and poverty. That is why there is more than the usual percentage of criminal eccentricity—the high rate of incest, for example (G. Lewis 1963:339).

Boys, on the other hand, wear only a short shirt, often until they go to school, and the exposed genitals are manipulated and admired to develop *machismo*. At an early age the boy is encouraged to express *machismo* through aggression, freedom of movement, feats of strength, verbal and mechanical skills, sexual prowess, the defense of his honor and that of his family, responsibility for his sister's virtue and his mother's good name, refusal to do "women's work," gambling, and drinking.

The girl is trained for the less complex role of subordination and submission. She must be chaste, docile, adept at domestic tasks and child-rearing, hardworking, clean, and ready to sacrifice herself for her family. Her toilet training is more severe, and her temper tantrums are quickly and decisively suppressed. She is much less indulged than her brother, but is treated more gently and affectionately because she is considered to be more delicate. She is carefully supervised in all her activities outside the home, especially in relation to men. She is trained consistently, continuously, and clearly for her adult role.

The boy, however, encounters inconsistency, discontinuity and frustration when he tries to perform the contradictory roles the culture prescribes. He, too, must be obedient, but since he is more indulged and encouraged to be aggressive, he is less obedient and therefore punished more often and more severely than the girl. He has a closer and more dependent relationship with his mother, but as a male he must be independent and dominant. *Machismo* requires proof of sexual con-quest, but access to the carefully guarded girls in many of the rural areas is difficult. Since sex is viewed as being essential to the male and he can rarely afford a prostitute, he is usually married by the time he is 18. And when he marries, the greatest obstacles prevent him from being a good provider, upon which male primacy in the family ultimately rests.

Everywhere rural children are trained to show *respeto* at a very early age. Learning this value regulates their relationships with all social superordinates, with their parents, their *compadres* and kin, and with older people.

Tables 6.1–6.4 show the variations among the rural subcultures in socioeconomic status, religion, ritual kinship, the nuclear and extended families, and child rearing.

Sociocultural Variables and Stresses

According to Steward, the most thoroughly adjusted groups in Puerto Rico are the two extremes of the class hierarchy:

the insular upper class who . . . have made their cultural choice, and . . . the laboring proletariat, for example at Canamelar [the corporation-owned sugar plantations on the south coast], whose roles and statuses are so in-escapably fixed that no choice is possible (1956:502).

But migration *is* a choice open to the workers in the sugarcane, and the extent of migration testifies to their lack of adjustment. Moreover, the *agregados* on the privately owned sugar *haciendas* have even lower status than the unionized proletariat on the south coast, but the pro-letariat seems to be much better adjusted than the *agregados,* and the difference in the degree of adjustment seems to result from factors other than lack of choice.

The degree of adjustment among adults is frequently reflected by the child-rearing practices of the group. The range of child-rearing practices of the five rural subcultures appears to constitute a "stress" continuum, with the south coast proletarian and the coffee *jíbaro* at the pole of least stress on the child as he is enculturated, and the sugar *agregado* at the opposite pole of greatest stress.

Yet the lifeways of the proletarian and the coffee *jíbaro* are at oppo-site poles on the folk-urban continuum. The land is of utmost impor-tance to the *jíbaro;* the proletarian has no land at all. The *jíbaro's* life is the most traditional; the proletarian's life is the least traditional. The *jíbaro* is the least involved in the cash economy; the proletarian works

Table 6.1—Variant Patterns and Values of the Rural Subcultures: Economic

	Coffee Highlands[1]	Tobacco Highlands	Sugar Haciendas	Sugar Farms North Coast	Sugar Farms South Coast
Landownership; Type and Size of Farm	family-owned; large: Spanish; small: Puerto Rican; also tobacco	mainly small and medium; family-owned; also mixed crops	medium; family-owned; monocrop	very large; government cooperative; functions to provide work	very large; corporation-owned; monocrop
Type of Labor and Returns	subsistence sharecropping; cash, perquisites; wage labor; exchange labor, small farms	cash-crop share-cropping; wage labor	wage labor; cash, perquisites; seasonal	unskilled wage labor includes women; seasonal; unionized; subsistence plots	unskilled wage labor; seasonal; strongly unionized
Employer-Employee Relations	traditional, hierarchical, personal	hierarchical, personal, somewhat commercial	traditional, hierarchical, personal	cash-based, impersonal	cash-based, impersonal
Subsidiary Economic Activities for Labor	seasonal migration; labor exchange	seasonal migration for wage laborer	gambling, making and selling bootleg rum	fishing, crabbing, sand hauling, stone quarrying	fishing, crabbing
Mobility for *jíbaro*	large farms grow larger; small farms, smaller; cash accumulation very difficult	cash accumulation possible by sharecropper for land purchase	very limited; only through gambling and migration	limited; mainly through gambling and migration	very limited; only through gambling and migration

[1]Data for this and the following three tables came from the following sources: Landy (1965), Manners (1956), Mintz (1956, 1960), Padilla-Seda (1956), Steward (1956), E. Wolf (1956), K. Wolf (1952).

Table 6.2—Variant Patterns and Values of the Rural Subcultures: Sociocultural

	Coffee Highlands	Tobacco Highlands	Sugar *Haciendas*	Sugar Farms North Coast	Sugar Farms South Coast
Major Goals of *jíbaro*	to retain farm	to buy a farm	migration to mainland	to leave the sugarcane	to leave the sugarcane
Religion	strongly Catholic, magic and witchcraft, saint cult	recreational aspects of Catholicism	some children attend Evangelical Church	Pentecostal, magic, witchcraft, saint cult	Pentecostal; religion not very important
Education	mediated by landowner, nonfunctional	good facilities, extensively used for upward mobility	valued for occupational improvement	valued for prestige, practical use, migration	valued if it removes children from sugarcane
Health and Medicine	folk theories and medicine	extensive use of clinics and doctors	folk theories and medicine; injections valued	folk theories and medicine; curer used for illness	folk and modern medicine; extensive use of clinics
Attitudes toward Deviance	aggression and physical defects accepted	emotional and mental deviants at home; aggression not accepted	"loco" and physical deviance accepted, but ridiculed		pity for helplessness
Valued Attributes	hard work, competence, cooperation, responsibility, thrift, hospitality	hard work, individual effort, independence, thrift, frugality, conformism	political connections, conformism	efficiency, responsibility	hard work, competence, group solidarity, individual autonomy, hospitality

Table 6.3—Variant Patterns and Values of the Rural Subcultures: Ritual Kinship and Family

	Coffee Highlands	Tobacco Highlands	Sugar *Hacienda*	Sugar Farms North Coast	Sugar Farms South Coast
Ritual Kinship, *Compadrazgo*	reinforces reciprocal inter-class, intraclass, neighbor, kin, relatives	intraclass; used for minor help	intraclass; secularized and weakened	reinforces intraclass relations, but attenuating	reinforces union and political affiliations; prevents worker competition
Extended Family	strongly coop-erative in exchange of labor, favors, hospitality	weak obligations	partially dis-integrated; less respect and support for aged	weak obligations	strong network of obligations and social relations; very important for children
Marriage	religious; arranged in connection with land ownership; stable	generally stable, religious and civil; a fourth, consensual	a fourth religious; half, civil; about a fourth, consensual	often consensual and unstable	predominantly consensual
Nuclear Family	patrilineal, large	patrilineal; large; nuclear family important	patrilineal, large	matrilineal, matricentric, matrinymic, average 3 children	matrilineal, large
Conjugal Relations	husband, authoritarian, not violent; wife, subservient, resentful	husband, authoritarian, sometimes abusive; wife, subordinate	husband, authoritarian, abusive; wife, subordinate, resentful	husband helps with chores; egalitarian	husbands help with children; egalitarian

Table 6.4—Variant Patterns and Values of the Rural Subcultures: Child Rearing

	Coffee Highlands	Tobacco Highlands	Sugar *Haciendas*	Sugar Farms North Coast	Sugar Farms South Coast
Affection	much, from parents, kin	for babies	for babies	from parents	much, from parents, extended family and neighbors
Aggression	controlled	tolerated in nuclear family	punished	controlled	controlled
Cooperation	stressed, in extended network		enforced	responsible for siblings	stressed, in extended network; sharing
Experimentation	encouraged		discouraged; dependence encouraged	moderate	encouraged; emotional independence strong
Frustration	baby permitted to feed only briefly	unfulfilled promises	unfulfilled promises		
Obedience	not enforced	enforced	enforced	stressed	not enforced
Punishment	beatings rare	beating, ego-deflating, teasing, mocking, threats of abandonment	beating, ego-deflating, threats: supernatural, environmental, castration	beating rare; ridicule	beating rare
Respeto	stressed	enforced	enforced	stressed	for *compadres*
Sex	discussed by women before children		sex "dirty"; masturbation prohibited	not discussed	free discussion; masturbation accepted
Toilet Training	not enforced	enforced by scolding, urging	enforced by scolding, beating	not enforced	not enforced

only for cash. The *jíbaro* is the most orthodox in religion; the proletarian is the most indifferent to religion. The *jíbaro* is the most concerned about legal marriage; the proletarian has the highest rate of consensual union. The *jíbaro's* family is strongly patrifocal; the proletarian's family tends to be matrifocal. The *jíbaro* is most authoritarian; the proletarian, most egalitarian. In the coffee highlands the *jíbaros* are mainly white; on the south coast the proletarians are generally black or mulatto.

However, the two subcultures are linked by a strong network of relationships, encompassing the extended family, neighbors, and class members, in which *compadrazgo* figures prominently. The adult's security and adjustment, which redound to the benefit of the child, derive from this network. "By making the adults in the social environment more interdependent and secure, *compadrazgo* gives to the child himself, even if a little indirectly, a firmer, more organized world" (Mintz 1956:388).

The obligations upon which this network of relationships rests are debilitated in the other rural subcultures. The tobacco *jíbaro* treats them lightly lest they hamper him in his drive for upward mobility. The north coast *jíbaro* makes effective use neither of his kin nor of the union. The sugar *agregado's* kinship ties disintegrate as he competes for scarce employment. In the rural areas where welfare benefits are minimal, only the strong extended family provides a modicum of security. Competition is therefore very threatening in the rural subcultures which no longer place high value on *compadrazgo* and the extended family. But in the coffee highlands and the south coast, *compadrazgo* is a stronger force than competition and reduces its impact.

Since the tobacco *jíbaro* is accorded respect only to the extent that he is successful in acquiring land, he hurries the child toward the achievement of those adult skills which will ensure his success. In his extreme poverty, the sugar *agregado* receives respect only in his home. This respect is a fictitious label for the subservience and fear he exacts from his wife and children, and duplicates the deference and humility he must display to his superordinates.

Relatively isolated in a punitive and threatening world, the sugar *agregado* and tobacco *jíbaro* transmit this image of the universe to the child as they enculturate him by physical punishment, ego-deflation and threats, insisting at the same time that he show them respect. The child's dependency, reinforced by an inculcated fear of the supernatural and the physical environment, is rejected, as he grows older, by his parents who engendered it in the first place. The child, in his turn, vents his humiliations, frustrations and hostility upon others who are helpless and vulnerable.

Since male dominance rests on the man's ability to be a good provider, a role almost impossible to fulfill, the universe is threatening and
insecure in all the rural subcultures. But the buffer in the coffee highlands and on the south coast is the network of interdependencies, which
are maintained by cooperation, generosity and hospitality, values which
receive major emphasis in child rearing. In the coffee highlands siblings
feel great responsibility for one another and the *jíbaro* teaches appreciation of human effort by the extensive use of praise. On the south
coast, sharing with siblings is pervasive, and the children are permitted
personal autonomy and emotional independence. In neither subculture
is the child hurried to maturity. In both he finds his way by imitation
and experimentation, helped by *cariño,* affection, another traditional
Puerto Rican value.

The two subcultures illustrate the effective operation of "social feedback" (Wiener 1954:50). Unconditional respect for the individual arises
out of the network of extensive relationships, regardless of the negative
attitudes of the wider society. The man who receives respect which is
not contingent on achievement and success has *dignidad,* intrinsic dignity. This man respects his child in the same way he is respected, and
the child, in turn, respects his parents and the community. Respect,
originating in the community, is directed back to the community.

But in the subcultures of the tobacco *jíbaro,* the sugar *agregado* and,
to some extent, the north coast proletarian, respect is enforced on the
parent, who enforces it on the child. Respect which is contingent on
achievement is conspicuous by its absence when it cannot be enforced.
Lack of respect also operates in social feedback from and to the community, mediated by adult and child. Lack of respect, or disrespect,
provokes anxiety and hostility, which must be repressed. Both anxiety
and hostility are associated with stuttering.

Certain attitudes toward speech in the subcultures which enforce
respect upon the child reflect their general child-rearing values. Respect
toward adults requires that the child "be seen and not heard." Children
must be quiet in the presence of adults, especially when the father is
eating, and they interrupt adult conversation at their peril. At the same
time verbal proficiency is required of the Puerto Rican *macho.* The
expectation that a man will be verbally quick and witty after he has
been trained to repress speech constitutes a major speech discontinuity,
which is undoubtedly a factor in the development of stuttering.

Moreover, children who in the presence of adults are forced to curb
most of their natural impulses, including the desire to communicate by
speech, often express violent and cruel aggression in their absence. This
is illustrated by the activities of children in a peasant community in the

southwest of the island when they are released from the severe restraints imposed upon them at home and in school:

these repressed children, quiet and shy at home in front of adults . . . broke into wild games when away from them. . . . Children threw stones at animals. . . . They called each other names . . . including stammerer (gago) . . . or any other name derived from a physical characteristic or from any social situation evaluated as ridiculous or embarrassing to the individual. . . . Other games operating as hostility-releasing activities for children were calling names to old people, drunks, idiots and other handicapped persons (Seda-Bonnilla 1958:77).

Comparing the Puerto Rican rural subcultures with the stuttering and nonstuttering societies, described earlier, the family patterns and child-rearing practices of the tobacco *jíbaro* and the *hacienda agregado* appear to be strikingly similar, in many respects, to those of the stuttering societies, the "tough" cultures. The values of the coffee *jíbaro* and the south coast proletarian, on the other hand, resemble those of the non-stuttering societies, the "easy" cultures. What happens to these differing values when the rural migrant acculturates in the slums of San Juan and New York?

CHAPTER 7

The Migrants in San Juan

The first surge of migration reached San Juan during the depression of the 1930s, when thousands of starving peasants went to the cities in search of work. The second migratory stream was a concomitant of insular industrialization and the decline in agriculture, particularly after World War II. In 1930 about 260,000 Puerto Ricans were employed in agriculture and about 98,000 in manufacturing (Perloff 1950:401). By 1957 industry had replaced agriculture as the major source of insular income, and by 1964, 139,000 people worked in agriculture, compared with 327,000 in nonagricultural industry.

Between 1930 and 1960 the population of Greater San Juan increased by two-thirds, and by 1962 it had grown to more than 600,000. "Most of its new residents come directly from agricultural villages or isolated farms, without intervening stages" (Caplow, Stryker, and Wallace 1964:3, 6).

From the time it was founded, early in the sixteenth century, San Juan has been the military, administrative, political, and intellectual center of Puerto Rico. The city has vast disparities in wealth, ranging from poverty just short of starvation to enormous affluence. Culturally it is a hybrid of Hispanic and North American traits. Architecturally and socially it is undergoing rapid change "under the impact of migration, slum clearance, a housing boom, highway development, the continued expansion of tourist facilities and the rapid progress of industrialization" (Caplow et al. 1964:32).

The San Juan urban area is divided into fifty-eight *barrios*,[1] ranging in size from 12 to 300 acres and containing from 375 to 70,000 people.

---

[1] Throughout Latin America the social unit is the *barrio*, something between an autonomous district and a census tract.

Some *barrios* "are almost nations in themselves, having a local dialect and an aversion to strangers" (Caplow et al. 1964:31). The people of San Juan are a mixture of Caucasoid, Negroid, and American Indian. Their median age is twenty-three, which is more than ten years younger than the urban median on the mainland, and they average 7.9 years of education.

The Culture of Poverty

The majority of the rural migrants in San Juan share some or all of the characteristics of the culture of poverty. Although the culture of poverty is widespread in Puerto Rico, it is by no means exclusively Puerto Rican. It often develops during a transitional period when a stratified social system, such as feudalism, is changing to capitalism, or when technology is developing rapidly in an agricultural society. The culture of poverty arises in societies with the following elements:

a cash economy, wage labor and production for profit; a persistently high rate of unemployment and underemployment for unskilled labor; low wages; the failure to provide social, political and economic organization, either on a voluntary basis or by government imposition, for the low-income population; . . . the existence of a set of values in the dominant class which stresses the accumulation of wealth and property, the possibility of upward mobility and thrift, and explains low economic status as the result of personal inadequacy or inferiority (O. Lewis 1965:xliv).

Those who become members of the culture of poverty are the lower strata which were already partially or wholly isolated from the social mainstream before it began to change. But the condition of poverty does not necessarily breed the culture of poverty. A simple preliterate society, poor in natural resources or technology, may have a more integrated and satisfying culture than that of many rural and urban slums. Nor is the culture of poverty generally widespread in "socialist, fascist and in highly developed capitalist societies with a welfare state" (O. Lewis 1965:1). Despite the considerable poverty in the United States, only about 20 percent of the population may be said to live in the culture of poverty because of the high aspirations in all sectors, and the advanced level of literacy, technology, and the mass media.

Oscar Lewis points out that people in the culture of poverty everywhere share "similarities in family structure, interpersonal relations, time orientation, value systems, spending patterns," and in their minimal participation in the principal social institutions. "A relief system which barely keeps people alive" only perpetuates "both the basic poverty and the sense of hopelessness." But when the poor become active members of trade unions or of any movement, "be it religious, pacifist or revolutionary," which gives them hope and promotes solidarity with a larger social institution, "the psychological and social core of the culture of poverty" is destroyed (1965:xliii, xlv-xlvi, xlviii).

Slum-dwellers who have stable residence, pay low and fixed rents, are united in kinship networks, or are members of organizations that maintain controls or obtain improvements, approach an integrated village in community spirit. But such conditions are absent in most rural and urban slums, where people are perpetually on the brink of crisis because of chronic unemployment, underemployment and low wages. These people depend on loans from neighbors and moneylenders. They pawn personal belongings, and buy small quantities of food whenever they have money. They use the culture of poverty to adapt to a marginal socioeconomic status, to cope with the feelings of hopelessness and despair which overwhelm them when they realize how unlikely they are to achieve success in terms of the dominant values and goals.

The people in the culture of poverty may lay claim to middle-class values, but rarely live by them. The high incidence of consensual unions, broken families, and matrifocal households are aspects of the culture of poverty throughout the world, in societies that have no history of slavery, and in urban as well as rural areas. Men who are in a chronic state of economic insecurity avoid the expenses involved in a legal union and probable divorce. Women refuse to be tied down "to men who are immature, punishing and generally unreliable." They feel that a consensual union "gives them some of the freedom and flexibility that men have, . . . a stronger claim on their children, . . . exclusive rights to . . . any property they may own" (O. Lewis 1965:xlvi).

According to Oscar Lewis, once the culture of poverty comes into being, it tends to perpetuate itself because of the effects on children.

By the time slum children are age six or seven they have usually absorbed the basic values and attitudes of their subculture and are not psychologically geared to take full advantage of changing conditions or increased opportunities which may occur in their lifetime (1965:xlv).

The culture of poverty has positive aspects. The people are oriented to the present and freely express sensuality, spontaneous impulses, and the desire for adventure "which is often blunted in the middle-class future-oriented man." Fatalism and a low level of aspiration tend to reduce frustration. Hostility is not repressed. "They tend to accept themselves as they are, and do not indulge in soul-searching or introspection." They often share food and clothing generously with the homeless and the ill (O. Lewis 1965:li, lii).

On the whole, however, the culture of poverty "does not provide much support or long-range satisfaction." It encourages mistrust, which "tends to magnify helplessness and isolation." In fact, "the poverty of culture is one of the crucial aspects of the culture of poverty" (O. Lewis 1965:lii).

Socioeconomic Status of the Migrants

The migrants bring to San Juan a rural heritage that includes extreme poverty, employment at a very early age, lack of education, serious family problems, broken homes, a pattern of violence, and poor physical and mental health. Respect and support for the aged began to decline before the migrants left the rural areas. Gambling has for centuries prevailed among all classes throughout the island. Folk patterns of religion and recreation were corroded by the mass media long ago. In the small, crowded rural huts children become aware of parental sexual relations at a very early age. The matrifocal family is a feature of the mountain towns and the coast, and polygyny and consensual unions transcend class lines. "The pattern of free unions and multiple spouses was not limited to the poor. It has been a widespread pattern among wealthy rural families" (O. Lewis 1965:xxviii).

Although increased stress is a concomitant of migration to the city, migrants with ample financial resources are protected from the severe dislocations of those who are poor. Perhaps the major stresses derive from industrialization, which may destroy old cultural values without replacing them by new meaningful integrations. But industrialization may simply accelerate processes which had already begun in the rural areas, such as the disorganization of the community, "the rural depopulation and cycles of migration that have created in Puerto Rico . . . the vast disease of urban rootlessness" (G. Lewis 1963:237).

The *jíbaro* comes to San Juan because he is seasonally employed, underpaid, undernourished, has little or no opportunity for advancement or choice of occupation, or because he can no longer endure his semifeudal dependence on the *hacendado*. Occasionally he migrates so that his children will get a better education, but generally he is in search of higher pay and greater vocational opportunity. However, "the son of a peasant in Puerto Rico has significantly lower chances for mobility into nonmanual occupations than the son of any other manual worker" (Tumin and Feldman 1961:444).

The *jíbaro* generally finds himself in Class V, the lowest of the five socioeconomic classes in San Juan. This class, which comprises 67 percent of the total San Juan population, consists mainly of unskilled and semiskilled workers, two-thirds with no more than four years of education (Rogler and Hollingshead 1965:49). Although San Juan offers a greater variety of occupations than the rural areas, few provide economic security for the migrants. They become factory workers, subject to discharge during slack periods; pick-and-shovel construction laborers and longshoremen, working part time and seasonally; service workers, affected by the vagaries of the tourist trade. A few are artisans, mainly masons and carpenters. Some are pushcart peddlers or run tiny stores in their homes.

Between 1940 and 1960, per capita income quintupled in Puerto Rico. But even in 1960 it reached only $677 (G. Lewis 1963:170). Thus very many Puerto Ricans were still extremely poor, and in San Juan the poorest were the people in Class V. Their median weekly family income in the late 1950s was $26; median weekly per capita income, $5; median daily per capita income, 71 cents (Rogler and Hollingshead 1965: 51). Class V people live in the slums, where four out of five persons come from the rural areas of the island (O. Lewis 1965:xxxv).

In the early 1950s the insular government embarked on a large-scale program to clear slums and build housing projects. "The era of explosive growth in San Juan has been succeeded by an era of intensive rebuilding" (Caplow et al. 1964:23). Whole *barrios* of slums were eliminated, but this was "barely sufficient to offset the natural increase of the slum population and the continued pressure of rural migration."

It will come as a shock to many Puerto Ricans who have watched their government's gigantic efforts at slum clearance in recent years to realize that, although the growth of the Slum Belt has been checked, only trifling progress has been made toward its removal. The decline of the slum population has recently averaged less than one-half of one per cent per year—a rate that, if continued, would give the Slum Belt two centuries more of existence (Caplow et al. 1964:228).

More than three-fourths of Class V people live in shantytowns, public housing projects, and slums. The remainder live in semirural *barrios* beyond the urban limits, which differ from urban slums mainly in being less crowded. These types of neighborhood are basically one-class segregations.

All too many community studies have mistaken one-class or two-class segregations . . . for communities. But the class is only part of a society; its culture only part of a larger order and civilization; its false community, only a segregation (Arensberg 1961:257).

The segregation of Class V people is particularly marked by "the rise of a dual educational system, with one education for the children of the middle class and one for the children of the poorer groups" (G. Lewis 1963:464). The enrollment of so many middle- and upper-class children in private and parochial schools has led to the demand that the private school be abolished as "an instrument of social, economic, racial and religious discrimination" (G. Lewis 1963:464).

Religion and recreation are also segregated on class lines. While once all classes celebrated the religious festivals together, now they celebrate them separately and differently. For recreation the middle and upper classes attend American movies, and the lower classes go to the less expensive movies made in Madrid and Mexico City.

Twenty percent of Class V marriages are consensual, compared with 10 percent in Class IV, and with the predominantly civil or religious marriages in the first three classes (Rogler and Hollingshead 1965:52). Moreover, the percentage of consensual unions among the lower classes tends to increase over time. "As members of the lower classes have broken up their marriages and gone on to new ones, some who were previously married in a legal union have now gone into consensual unions instead" (Tumin and Feldman 1961:253).

When the migrant arrives in San Juan he generally goes to a shanty-town where he is integrated into a network of relationships by relatives and friends who are already established, and who orient the newcomer to urban life, help him find a job and a place to live, and also help him build a house. But the shantytown imposes a different life-style than the housing project, especially on family structure and child-rearing patterns.

The Shantytown

Slums are old residential areas near the center of a city, where the buildings have been "converted from their original use to tenements housing many times their appropriate occupancy" (Icken 1962:1). A shantytown, on the other hand, is built on the periphery of a city, on marginal land unfit for residential or commercial use. When a slum is being cleared, useable material is immediately picked up before the debris can be removed and is rebuilt into a shanty.

In the middle 1950s, about 150,000 people in San Juan were living in shantytowns. "One of the world's most spectacular slums, La Perla," which has an informal list of people waiting to move in, "represents the last step before the upwardly mobile enter the world of lower middle-class respectability" (Caplow et al. 1964:35, 78). Another beach slum,

La Esmeralda, is known "as the home of murderers, drug addicts, thieves and prostitutes" (O. Lewis 1965:xxxiii).

"The largest slum in the world, El Fanguito, 'the little mud hole'" (Back 1962:9), is typical of most, for aside from those that shelter an unusually large number of social deviants, shantytowns do not differ substantially from one another. "El Fanguito" is, in fact, the name of only one of the eight *barrios* which stretch for more than 5 miles along the meandering dead water leading into the Martin Pena Channel, for many years the central sewer of the city. In the 1950s, El Fanguito contained 86,000 people, with a median age of eighteen years, the lowest in San Juan. "Welfare cases, infant mortality, tuberculosis, pneumonia, delinquency and other indices of social pathology, are much higher than anywhere else in the urban area" (Caplow et al. 1964:41).

Although the land is public property, the government does not try to dislodge shantytown residents, who form a substantial proportion of the urban electorate, except during slum clearance. Since the shanty owners are compensated for the loss of their homes during slum clearance, legal ownership of the shanties is tacitly acknowledged, and the purchase and sale of shanties are legal transactions.

All houses are built on piles to raise them above the frequent floods in the area, but so great is the demand for land that houses are built over the waters of the channel itself. Not only do they vibrate at high tide, but many can be reached only by a series of planks laid over the mud. The average density is greater than 90 persons per net residential acre (Caplow et al. 1964:56). By the end of the 1950s, the shantytowns had no sewage system, and in some *barrios* water was supplied by only one public faucet. Since garbage was not collected, it was thrown into the channel.

But over the years the residents have obtained police and fire protection, and many shantytowns have health and welfare services, elementary schools, inside electricity, running water, and wooden sidewalks.

it is a well-known fact that the eradication of urban slum areas like the San Juan eyesores . . . has been slowed down by the willingness of politicians to see a source of electoral strength in obtaining essential services like light, water and improved streets for the slum poor (G. Lewis 1964:204).

However, most streets are not yet lit or paved. In dry weather the air is full of dust from passing traffic, and in rainy weather the streets turn to mud and are sometimes impassable.

A shantytown is a modified folk culture. Although the more affluent families move to higher-priced neighborhoods and others move to housing projects, the population is constantly being replenished by new migrants with rural values and folkways. But the shantytown residents "are geared to the organic functioning of a society which.. . . . is dominated by nonfolk" (Foster 1953:170), and the folk culture is affected by a number of influences.

The shantytown dweller is a member of his *barrio,* of the urban proletariat, and of the city. But he is first a member of his *barrio,* "and only secondarily a member of the urban proletariat." His membership in the metropolis comes third and is the weakest link "in terms of interaction and identification" (Icken 1962:134). When they are not at their jobs, shantytown residents spend most of their time in their own neighborhood. They are outgoing and friendly, and show little distrust of strangers. "They live amid constant noise from radios, juke boxes and television sets, and spend a great deal of time in the stores and bars, where they drink and play dominoes" (O. Lewis 1965:xxxiii).

In the integrated shantytown men cooperate to improve conditions and to maintain and regulate social controls. The more affluent gain prestige by helping the indigent and often share utilities with people who are too poor to afford them.

The pattern of sharing guarantees . . . a certain minimum degree of security. No one is likely to starve where there are neighbors and relatives to help, though many undoubtedly go hungry and suffer from malnutrition (Icken 1962:89).

The integrated neighborhood plays the part of the extended family in rearing the child, for "the intensity of socializing among adults carries over to the children" (Icken 1962:183), who are included in the family's social life, as in the rural areas. Women help each other during pregnancy, after childbirth, and with child care. Neighborhood children play together and often marry childhood friends. People of all ages play baseball, the favorite sport, and "many of the most famous players on professional teams are persons who rose from the ranks of the rural or urban lower class" (Icken 1962:134).

The typical shantytown, however, is not well integrated. Of 25 *barrios* randomly selected for a study on the intensity of neighboring in San Juan, the two shantytown *barrios,* located in the Martin Pena Channel area, were very poorly integrated. Interfering factors were overcrowding, very poor facilities, rumors of slum clearance, religious differences, crime and delinquency, hopelessness about upward mobility. In one shantytown *anomie* was more marked than in any of the other 24 *barrios* in the study.

Twenty years of urban residence finds them . . . perhaps as badly off as they were in the country, with hope for improvement fading. There is not much left to expect but more filth, insults, fights and misery (Caplow et al. 1964:93).

Shantytown workers do not identify strongly as class members because the union movement, the usual means of gaining working-class identification, "is weak, disunited, immature" in Puerto Rico. Since union leaders are frequently "labor lawyers often unscrupulous in their search for handsome fees," working men believe they can exercise greater control over union officials in small unions that represent individual trades. In the larger unions, most rank and file members tend to be apathetic for "both at the local and territorial levels the union organizations have become so much the instrument of labor politicians in their struggle for political spoils" (G. Lewis 1963:229). In addition, when national unions, controlled on the mainland, negotiate with employers in Puerto Rico, they often ignore the local unions on whose behalf they are ostensibly negotiating.

Moreover, the important contribution of mainland capital to the growing industrialization of Puerto Rico is based on tax exemptions and low labor costs, and "it is not easy to unionize a factory whose owners can threaten to leave the island if labor costs increase." According to the AFL-CIO, the differences in wage rates between the mainland and the island have made Puerto Rico "a 'refuge' for unconscionable employers" (G. Lewis 1963:229, 220).

Through his union affiliations, which are strengthened by ritual kinship, the proletariat identify more strongly as class members on the south coast than in the city. The workers in the cane do much the same kind of labor in the same place at the same time, but the men living in the shantytown disperse throughout the city for their jobs.

In a society where unemployment and underemployment are chronic, and labor unions are weak, the traditional pattern of dominance-submission between employer and employee is reenforced. A recent study showed that the Puerto Rican lower-class man found it almost impossible to play "the role of a worker asking for a raise, where the only solution was to criticize the boss severely."

The difficulty of criticizing the boss fits well with the somewhat authoritarian social structure in Puerto Rico. When the test was given to a population of similar economic background in Chicago, no difficulty of this kind was encountered (Back 1962:22).

A very wide range of income and living standards prevails in the one-class shanty town. In Icken's sample population, 15 percent, mainly skilled workers, earned as much as $3000 a year, and with more than one wage earner in a household, family income sometimes reached $5000. About a fourth of the families earned less than $1000. When no one was employed, families depended on subsidiary economic activities and welfare, and income might go below $500 (Icken 1962:92, 104). As in the rural areas, men made illegal rum and sold tickets for the illegal lottery, both of which are very risky enterprises.

At times it seems that about the only thing that holds the various social classes together is the hope of making a killing in the state lottery or in the illegal *bolita* game. The taste for gambling, indeed, appears to be one facet of general consumption habits that has remained constant throughout the last two decades of . . . change. . . . It is clearly a living inheritance from the Spanish period (G. Lewis 1963:258).

When the men are unemployed, women may work part time in a laundry, take care of upper-class children, or engage in folk enterprises. They grow herbs and sell them for use in folk medicines. They sell roast chestnuts and ices from their homes. They may raise a pig or chickens for meat and eggs for the family, as well as for sale.

The houses in a shantytown are generally made of scrap material, under which a solid foundation develops in time by the accretion of garbage and rocks under the floor. The one-room shacks are improved as resources permit and a few end up as three-bedroom houses, with a living room, a kitchen, and a flush toilet emptying its wastes into the channel. But most houses have only one bedroom, with a latrine and a shower improvised in a closet at the back. "The extent of overcrowding can be judged from the fact that . . . there is an average of 3.42 persons per bedroom . . . and 2.15 persons per bed" (Icken 1962:70). Nevertheless, shanty ownership is a basic form of security, for it provides shelter for the family.

Even those who can afford it do not buy expensive furniture because of the hazards of termites, the constant dampness, fire, flooding, and hurricanes. But in 1960, one out of every eight people in the shantytowns owned a car (Caplow et al. 1964:58); there is a radio in almost every house, and many families have refrigerators and television sets.

To look at the bizarre combination of squalid huts and television antennae in the fetid slums of *El Fanguito* and *La Perla* is to be made forcibly aware . . . of the distorted social values to which the struggle [la *lucha*, "the rat race"] is dedicated (G. Lewis 1963:258).

The food staple is rice and beans, but there is the same range in the quantity and quality of the diet as in housing. More money is spent for food than for any other item in the family budget, but uncertain income makes budgeting impossible.

The same kind of clothing is worn all year. However, it is considered imperative to buy children new outfits at the beginning of the school year, and they are sometimes kept out of school until parents can afford to clothe them properly. Although Puerto Rican women are usually skilled at sewing and could save money by making clothes for their families, disproportionately large amounts are spent on store-bought clothes. "The emphasis upon clothing and appearance . . . may . . . have been caused by inferiority feelings and reparative needs and by imitation of the Puerto Rican middle class, which stresses the importance of clothing" (O. Lewis 1965:xxxvii).

Considerable money is also spent for special events, such as graduations, church baptisms, and holidays, and, for the upwardly mobile, elaborate church weddings. These occasions serve to renew ties with near and distant relatives, *compadres* and friends. "Empty stomachs often accompany efforts to participate with splendor and affluence on these gala days" (Rogler and Hollingshead 1965:285).

In the city the traditional conjugal roles change and family life is often disrupted, for women can also find work in the factories and service industries. The husband, however, opposes such employment because it reflects on his ability to support the family, and the working wife's economic independence threatens his authority in the home. Usually a woman with small children does not go out to work, but in many families the woman is the principal breadwinner. When a man cannot obtain work over a long period, he may totally abdicate his responsibilities and desert his family. Or he may become abusive, and the woman will leave him and work to support the children. Thus economic instability contributes to marital instability.

Despite the greater economic independence of women in the shantytown, sex roles remain clearly differentiated. Even when the wife works outside the home she is responsible for the care of the family and the household. In addition to his primary work role, the man maintains and repairs the house and perhaps does the weekly marketing, but a woman can expect very little help from her husband, for doing "woman's work" subjects a man to ridicule.

In part it is the terror of ridicule that makes the Puerto Rican so conscious of respect. Both husband and wife believe that respect is a necessary prerequisite for love. "If a choice has to be made, 73 percent of the wives and 70 percent of the husbands prefer respect over love from their mates" (Rogler and Hollingshead 1965:267). But the value of *respeto* creates a communications barrier between husband and wife. They do not discuss sex and birth control, and the husband does not talk to his wife about his work, the amount of money he earns, and his social activities. A man gives his wife an allowance or doles out money when she needs it, but he rarely tells her how much money he keeps for himself.

The culture prescribes respect both for the good family man and for the *macho,* and the roles are in conflict. A man who drinks, gambles, and consorts with other women is a *macho,* but he deprives his family and shows a lack of respect for his wife. The traditionally *conforme* Puerto Rican woman deeply resents her husband's infidelity and this is another reason for leaving him. In fact, suspected and actual sexual infidelity are a major source of family disruption.

There is an overwhelming preoccupation with sex, the most frequent cause of quarrels. Sex is used to satisfy a great variety of needs—for children, for pleasure, for money, for revenge, for love, to express *machismo* . . . and to compensate for all the emptiness in their lives (O. Lewis 1965:xxvi).

With little communication between husband and wife, and few common interests besides the children, blood ties are much stronger than conjugal bonds. A woman makes every effort to live near her own relatives, especially her mother. In fact, as on the coast, the ability to count on her own kin is an important factor in a woman's independence. A woman looks to her children and the extended family for emotional support, help in the home, and economic assistance when she needs it.

Women prefer legal marriage, which makes the father responsible for the children's support and facilitates obtaining welfare. Lower-class women, however, are less likely to accept a distressing marriage than middle- and upper-class women. Lower-class women who break up a marriage have less to lose in economic support, and they are more self-reliant and better able to take care of themselves and their families without a husband's help. Also, "more than four times as many marriages in the lowest as in the highest class were dissolved because of death" (Tumin and Feldman 1961:254), which comes much earlier to those in poor physical and mental health.

Frequently it is the Puerto Rican men who are more interested in preserving the family and who resist their wives' attempts to separate. The women in the slums are more aggressive and violent than the men, and usually direct their aggression against the men.

The women continually deprecate them and characterize them as inconsiderate, irresponsible, untrustworthy and exploitative. . . . On the whole, the men seem to be more passive, dependent and depressed than the women (O. Lewis 1965:xxvi).

Welfare payments are pitifully inadequate in Puerto Rico. According to the *New York Times* of October 14, 1968 (p. 28), the average monthly payment was $24.50 for a family of four. Because of this, it is not unusual for women who support their families to enter into casual sexual liaisons. "The exchange of sexual services for support on a semipermanent basis is more common than outright prostitution in the shantytown" (Icken 1962:131). But prostitution is not rare.

For unskilled, often illiterate women, whose lives are a struggle for survival, prostitution is a tempting economic alternative which does not necessarily ostracize them from their neighbors or social group, and which does not represent as sharp a break from ordinary life as it does for middle-class women (O. Lewis 1965:xxx).

Despite the increase in conjugal stress, the man's role in the shantytown is paramount. He is the principal breadwinner in the majority of families, and he builds the house which shelters his wife and children. He also represents the family both in the neighborhood and in the larger society. In the integrated shantytown men have much more opportunity to demonstrate leadership qualities than in the rural community which is dominated by the *hacendado*.

While husband and wife do not value each other highly in the conjugal role, they have no doubts about the parental role. Children fulfill both sexes, and since they make little economic contribution in the shantytown, they are loved for themselves alone. As on the north coast, families have an average of three children, which may include those who are informally adopted in emergencies.

Despite their love of children, the practice of giving children to relatives, *compadres,* and neighbors is common among all classes in Puerto Rico, but widespread in the slums. While this practice gives a woman greater freedom of movement, its effects on the child are questionable. "Adult Puerto Ricans never think of this custom . . . as abandonment, but studies suggest that some children feel it as such" (O. Lewis 1965: xxix). And because of the preference for "whiteness," the darker-skinned child is often the one who is given away.

Sometimes a woman is forced to take into her home a child that her husband fathered with another woman, "not only during a previous marriage but during a casual liaison" (Icken 1962:174). However, most women treat these *hijos de crianza* in the same way as their own children.

Child rearing in the shantytown is a mixture of traditional and modern practices. Children are breast-fed until the next pregnancy, as in the rural areas, but bottles may also be used. "Diapers are seldom used for either sex, except in families consciously imitating middle-class standards" (Icken 1962:174). Traditional charms are still used to protect the baby against *mal de ojo,* and sex differentiation begins at a very early age, with modesty training for the girls. Children are usually baptized at home, church baptism being postponed until the family can afford the indispensable celebration.

Both men and women try to perpetuate the traditional roles, but the city itself forces change. "Pressures that impinge on a growing child are seen to be by-products of a horde of considerations that impinge upon the parents and influence their child-rearing practices" (Honigmann 1967:290).

Children are punished physically at an earlier age and more frequently in the shantytown than in the coffee highlands and on the coast. In the rural areas the father does not need to resort to beating his children to obtain respect and obedience, for his authority is unquestioned, and children are directly involved in important economic activities under parental surveillance. In San Juan, however, father and son have no working relationship, and parents present a model for physical violence which cannot be hidden from the children. Parents are affectionate with their children, but at the same time, reports Hazel Stanton, "they bang those kids against the wall . . . and they really beat them up" (1966:50).

Children's aggression is also much less strongly controlled in the shantytown than in the rural areas or in middle-class communities. "Fighting goes on from a very early age even among siblings regardless of sex" (Stanton 1966:20). Mothers are more accepting of verbal aggression against themselves, and parents are not as strict in controlling their children's disrespect. Nevertheless, *respeto* is still a basic value, even though it requires more frequent and severe punishment to be enforced.

Every blow aimed at him is accentuated by "para que cojas respeto" ("so that you will learn respect"), an exclamation often heard over the screeches and wails of a child even during a short visit to a slum or caserio [housing project] (Rogler and Hollingshead 1965:386).

Children prefer the mother to the father, who is away from home a great deal even when he is unemployed. In fact, mothers teach their children to depend on them and to distrust the father.

Girls become useful in the home at a very early age, and when mothers work, elder daughters assume full responsibility for all the children except the older brothers. Aside from running errands and trying to make money by doing odd jobs, boys are always with their friends and come home only for meals. The girl, like her mother, is central to the household. The boy is marginal to it, like his father, and many adolescent boys look to the peer group for a masculine model. However, in a number of shantytowns there is no separate adolescent subculture, and play groups include all ages. Boys remain a part of the family and of the neighborhood and, although the older generation has less authority than in the rural areas, children still show respect for adults. The father usually retains some control over his son, and when the father is absent, another male adult, usually a relative, acts as a father surrogate.

The behavior of the girl also changes in the shantytown. Girls still internalize the concept of virginity and generally do not have sexual relations until they reach the elopement stage because they are afraid they will become pregnant or "get a bad name." But sexual segregation is far less rigidly enforced in the shantytown than in the rural areas. Girls are not chaperoned, and there are more places where young people may meet. Girls are much more direct with men in the shantytown than in the highlands, and the dividing line between courtship and marriage is unclear, as in the coastal areas. They may marry total strangers who have picked them up, and "it is not unheard-of to be introduced for the first time to the spouse's family after a *fait accompli"* (Stanton 1966:30).

Getting and keeping a mate is a constant activity since many are looking to better their chances. . . . The non-virgin or previously married female also competes on a level not too different from that of the never married virgin (Stanton 1966:32).

Since unions are based on romantic love they are often short-lived. The spouse comes first when the couple has no problems, but when conflicts arise the blood relative is primary, for "few people would place their future in the hands of their husband or wife" (Stanton 1966:31).

As the *jíbaro* does not want his son to be a farm worker, so parents in the shantytown want to rid the children of the stigma of manual labor. They hope their children will become white-collar workers and professionals, but say the neighborhood prevents achievement and they themselves "do not have the economic and intellectual resources to help their children realize the aspirations they claim to have." Children are not rewarded for academic achievement or punished for lack of it. As in the rural areas, girls are taken out of school to help at home, and a boy who finds a job leaves school. Moreover, the value of *respeto,* which "demands that you stay in your place and behave according to your publicly recognized traditional status," is dysfunctional for upward mobility in an urban environment. Thus, "two-thirds of the children in school are behind in their grade placement; the boys, almost two years and the girls, almost three years" (Rogler and Hollingshead 1965:399, 408, 393). In the early 1960s, 66 percent of the young people between the ages of fourteen and nineteen "were school drop-outs, and about 20 percent of all those fourteen years of age or over were illiterate" (O. Lewis 1965:xxxvi).

Parents who work in industry, however, whether in rural or urban areas, and who have more than a minimal education, are more successful in implementing their aspirations for their children. A study of nine-to-thirteen-year-old boys in intact families of small farmers and factory workers in rural areas showed that factory fathers express affection for sons more openly and use physical punishment less often than farm fathers. Parents in the less educated factory group stressed obedience and conformity in school, and the sons did not incorporate values about educational achievement. But in the more educated factory families boys were responsible for chores at home, mothers often pressed for academic achievement, and fathers participated in their sons' activities and helped their children with school work. The fathers also encouraged children to fight for their rights and were more tolerant of aggression against parents. "The children of the factory-educated parents . . . are the ones who are most likely to . . . want to work for goals of social value and to make money" (Mussen 1966:182).

The attitudes and income of people with five or more years of schooling differ considerably from those with up to four years. "In San Juan, the most disproportionate gain in income is made in the transition from 1–4 to 5–8 years of education" (Tumin and Feldman 1961:63). But only about 28 percent of Class V adults in San Juan have completed five to eight years of school (Rogler and Hollingshead 1965:49).

However, the children of the rural migrants generally do achieve much more education than their parents. Although most of the parents have no more than three or four years of schooling, the children usually complete elementary school. More than half the young people in Icken's sample shantytown completed the eighth grade and more than 40 percent were attending high school (Icken 1962:188). And although women in the rural areas have even less education than men, "the studies on school drop-out show that boys do tend to drop out in larger proportions than girls" in the city.[2] Thus the children of the rural migrants move increasingly into the middle class.

Adolescents in the shantytown have severed their rural ties completely and have set their sights on the symbols of middle-class status—a high school education, a white-collar job, a home in an *urbanización* (new suburban sub-division). Some even hope to go to college and become teachers, nurses or engineers (Icken 1962:189).

The Public Housing Project

Not only does the rural migrant suffer culture shock from the process of urbanization and the new type of work he does in San Juan, but he is also dislocated by changes imposed by "public policy and economic evolution. . . . Highway development, industrial development, urban renewal, harbor improvements and the breakneck growth of public facilities displace thousands of families within the metropolitan area every year" (Caplow et al. 1964:3–4).

However, the Urban Renewal and Housing Corporation of the Commonwealth meets with considerable resistance from many of the families it displaces and seeks to relocate, despite its waiting list of tenants. "The events which the administrator calls 'slum clearance' and 'relocation' are seen by the people as loss of home and exposure to the hazards of a new way of life" (Back 1962:4). The "pathology of social fear in which the proletarian lives" comes to public attention "when, for example, slum dwellers refuse to move to new housing projects because of their fears of a new economic regimentation that the compulsory payment of rent brings to their mind" (G. Lewis 1963:485). Two-thirds of Back's sample of a hundred tenants stated that they had moved into the project "only because they were forced to do so." Ninety percent "would prefer their own solutions to a housing project" (1962:60, 65).

The shantytown dweller not only does not pay rent, in most cases, but he also often taps power lines and does not pay for electricity. The idea of paying both rent and the cost of electricity out of a low, irregular income creates the utmost anxiety, and is the primary reason for the resistance to moving into a housing project.

---

[2]Commonwealth of Puerto Rico, Department of Education, *The Puerto Rican Child in His Cultural Context*. Barranquitas: Commonwealth of Puerto Rico, Department of Education, 1966, p. 71. Mimeographed.

In addition, the shantytown resident strongly resents the prohibitions in housing projects. The rule against keeping domestic animals may deprive him of an important supplement to his income and diet. The rule against running a lunch counter or small shop in his home may deprive him of his total income. And the rule against overnight visitors deeply offends the migrant who is generally separated from the extended family when he leaves the shantytown. Furthermore, competition from so many low-income people in the project reduces the number of odd jobs available from the higher-income residents in the neighborhood.

Finally, the integrated shantytown gives its dwellers emotional and financial security. "Well-known neighbors moved to assist in emergencies and would allow credit to be established in the stores" (Back 1962:10). The very fact of home ownership is basic to the shantytown dweller's security.

In his housing preferences, the San Juanero belongs entirely to North America, not to Latin America or Europe. His preference for single family housing over multiple dwellings is overwhelming and cannot be satisfied by low-rise apartments (Caplow et al. 1964:229).

In 1954 about 8,000 families were living in housing projects, apartments for an additional 10,000 were being built, and relocation from twenty-five sites and twenty-one localities was in process (Back 1962:9). Moving into a project imposes great changes in living conditions, health, family structure, delinquency, class orientation, and social status.

In a country like Puerto Rico, the implications of a move to a housing project are tremendous. It means moving from small houses to apartment buildings, from wooden construction to concrete buildings, from squatters' rights to tenancy, from shifting day by day to planned administration. Thus it involves not only the connotations such a move would have in a city in the United States, but a further step in the process of urbanization as well (Back 1962:107).

The facilities of the housing projects are superior to those of the shantytown. The projects have well-lit, paved streets, sewerage, and electricity, and the apartments have separate kitchens and bathrooms. Health improves in the projects, particularly that of the children, who "show a much lower incidence of illnesses such as diarrhea, pneumonia, anemia and internal parasites" (Icken 1962:202). Since the apartments are generally larger than the shanties, fewer persons occupy a bed, although there may be as many persons per room. In the shantytown, status symbols derive from the condition and size of the house and the number of appliances; in the project, they derive from the quantity and quality of the furniture.

The project studied by Icken contained play space for young children and for several sports, enclosed areas for drying laundry and stacking garbage cans, a health center and medical dispensary, two nurseries, a milk station, a breakfast center for preschool children, a library, an elementary school, and a junior high school. Home economics courses were offered to women, and night classes were held for adults. The community center sponsored clubs for children, adolescents, and adults. The project was located close to a modern shopping center, a public park, and the beach. Although people had to pay cash at the supermarket, they could obtain credit from small merchants who drove their trucks illegally through the project area (1962:196).

According to Gordon Lewis, however, planners have generally failed "to provide adequate public facilities such as . . . playgrounds, parking areas, and community centers in the new housing developments." More than a fourth of the children in the city attended school for only half a day in the 1950s because of "the failure to provide enough schools to keep up with the pressing educational demands of the new communities spawned by the mass housing projects" (1963:203, 462).

Although the United States government contributed almost "$300 million in federally insured mortgages and nearly two-thirds the cost of all urban projects in the island," it did not receive public credit for this aid. The Federal Housing and Home Finance Agency has resented "this effort to make political capital out of American economic aid" (G. Lewis 1963:183).

The federal government also provides the architectural designs and sets the rules for administration and tenant selection. In selecting tenants, officials on the mainland ignored long-standing relationships in cohesive communities; initially they viewed the projects as transient housing for upwardly mobile lower-income people who would eventually move into private apartment houses or buy their own homes. But only a small minority of families, who rarely identify with the majority, use the projects as a springboard for change and upward mobility. Even though housing managers on the island are Puerto Rican and are educated in Puerto Rico, they are trained by mainland methods and philosophy. With its middle-class norms, project management tends to view the values and life patterns of the tenants as inferior, and has therefore "met with serious obstacles in its efforts to integrate families from shantytowns into a new way of life in public housing" (Icken 1962:192).

The people in Icken's sample project are physically separated from a working-class *barrio* by a major multilane expressway and by the rule that outsiders may not use project facilities. Their closest neighbors are upper-class people who are socially aloof and whose private homes are in striking contrast to the barracks-like project buildings, so that the tenants are "painfully aware of their low-status position in the larger society" (1962:205). Thus the project stands, an isolated segregation, the range of its one class considerably narrower than that of the shantytown.

The socioeconomic characteristics and family structure of project tenants differ markedly from those of shantytown residents. When slums are cleared, the oldest sites are generally the first to be demolished. But these are the sites of the best homes, owned by families with the highest income in the shantytown. These families generally consist of several wage-earning adults and few children. They strongly oppose the destruction of their homes and in any case rarely move into the projects. Those who do move into public housing are mainly the poorest families that are among the minority living in rented houses, usually the most dilapidated in the shantytown. These families tend to have younger household heads, one wage earner and several children. The majority have little hope of upward mobility, but they enjoy at least as good living conditions in public housing as those with higher incomes in the shantytown.

Although the mean educational level of both shantytown and project was the third grade, in Icken's sample populations, 21 percent of the project men were unemployed compared with 13 percent of the shantytown men (1962:211). In Back's sample populations, 40 percent of the tenants were laborers and service workers, compared with 20 percent in the shantytown; 29 percent of the project men were skilled and semiskilled, compared with 40 percent in the shantytown; 4 percent of the tenants had white-collar jobs, compared with about 10 percent in the shantytown (1962:30).

More women in the shantytown are regularly employed than in the project. Project women often work temporarily as domestics because they can more easily conceal this type of employment from management, as well as from the welfare agency, which cuts payments when family income increases. In Back's sample project the median annual family income was $776; in the shantytown, it was $1,448 (Back 1962: 30). Thus public housing defeats its professed aim of stimulating upward mobility.

Since the projects have a higher concentration of low-income families and a smaller number of families with higher incomes, they are much more homogeneous than the shantytowns. The smaller number of higher incomes is related to the fewer families with more than one wage earner, as well as to the fact that families with incomes higher than a certain level must move from the project, which is then deprived of a leadership core.

In Back's study, almost a third of the project families were broken, compared with about a fifth of the shantytown families (1962:30), for when the shantytown families move into the project, the men usually become even more marginal to the family. When a man gives up his shanty, he loses the principal means of protecting his family, his basic prop for authority in the family, and his independence from regimentation and external control. Since rent is based on income, all changes in job and income must be reported to management, which may check the information with the employer. The regular inspection of apartments for evidence of greater income in the form of new furniture or appliances is another invasion of family privacy.

"Twice as many project families are totally dependent on public welfare as families in the shantytown," Back says. The welfare worker has an important voice in decisions on family budgeting, and the father ceases to be the final authority on how income is spent. Since project managers and welfare workers are usually women, the man finds it humiliating to submit to a paternalism that uses women as its agents. He therefore yields to his wife his role of dealing with the outside world on behalf of the family, and her responsibility and authority increase.

Relocation in public housing is accompanied by the dispersal of friends and relatives throughout the city, and the absence of male friendships in the project is in striking contrast with male sociability in the shantytown. Men are not permitted to gather informally in the community room of the project to chat, have a drink, and play dominoes.

The project man is stripped of all the functions he performed in the shantytown except his purely economic function, the most precarious of all. Children in the project generally see the father "as a perpetually frustrated and inadequate little man, unrespected by his wife, dependent on employers, landlords, ward-heelers and bartenders for everything from job, credit and promotions, to getting the broken window fixed." Such a father finds it very difficult to maintain control over his son, and the son "is not going to find it easy himself to develop a mature personality" (Icken 1962:230). Thus in the project conjugal and generational bonds are further weakened, and the number of matrifocal families increases. When the father is absent, the mother finds it even more difficult to discipline the children, especially adolescent boys, who may leave school and refuse to work.

Lacking an integrated social network, men rely on management and the police to settle quarrels between neighbors and to control the behavior of young people. By its paternalistic policy, management produces a community "incapable of responsibility, expectant of unlimited care, resentful that all demands are not met, . . . and resentful also because of its own lack of independence" (Icken 1962:230). This resentment expresses itself in disaffection with the government and the Popular Party, to which the shantytown dwellers are loyal, and even more vehemently against management. Tenants who rarely cooperate with each other on any issue unite in their opposition to management.

The lack of tenant participation in the affairs of the project also results in many problems for management, such as nonpayment of rent, poor maintenance of apartments and grounds, vandalism, and juvenile delinquency. While juvenile delinquency increases mainly because of the loss of paternal authority in the home, the age-graded clubs in the project help to direct the adolescent to a peer group. The youth subculture "replaces the strong attachment to the family, and particularly to the mother, in the shantytown household," and it may develop into a gang which destroys property and bullies tenants. From the mass media adolescents learn to identify with American styles of dress and music rather than with Puerto Rican models, and some of the girls and boys adopt "the teenage courtship patterns of East Harlem" (Icken 1962:231, 233).

Icken represented the shantytown and the public housing project as opposite poles of integration. However, Caplow, et al. showed a range of integration among both shantytowns and projects. The two shantytowns in their study were poorly integrated, and one of the two projects was located in a *barrio* that illustrated a "tribal" pattern of neighboring.

There are few isolates . . . everyone knows everyone else and associates actively with nearly everyone else. The neighborhood is an extension of the family. It exerts continuous social influence and absorbs a large part of the free time and energy of its residents. There are no exclusive cliques (1964:73).

According to Caplow, et al., "people who have close relationships with their neighbors are more satisfied with their neighborhoods as places to live." Thus, many people who "live in neighborhoods considered 'squalid' and 'shocking' by outside observers, express a degree of satisfaction with their surroundings which borders on complacency." A well-integrated neighborhood, however, is not the only source of neighborhood satisfaction. Neighborliness appears to increase when society provides "a rising level of welfare," and adequate facilities within the building and the locality. The study found that "the relationship between bedroom density and moving intentions is spectacular." (Caplow et al. 1964:168, 197, 199, 203). Thus, residents of some projects are very satisfied with their neighborhoods.

The study revealed a tendency toward informal discrimination against nonwhites and non-Catholics; a homogeneous population is positively and significantly associated with neighboring intensity. A very important finding was the positive and significant correlation between neighboring intensity and every criterion of class position. "In San Juan, at least, the rich are better integrated into the urban network than the poor. Prosperity, *not* misery, likes company. Sociability declines as the need for support and assistance increases." However, the rural migrant appears to receive as much support in San Juan as he received in his village. The longer he stays in the city, the more acclimated he becomes and the greater the increase in "both the intensity and extensity of neighboring" (Caplow et al. 1964:224, 223).

Only 3.2 percent of the sample population studied by Caplow and associates showed "no neighboring." Compared with findings in studies on neighboring in American cities of similar size, "neighboring may be more intense in San Juan than in urban areas of the United States" (1964:158).

Although problems of segregation by color and ethnic origin exist in San Juan, they are much less severe than in most North American cities. Although juvenile delinquency is widespread and getting worse, no part of San Juan has the jungle atmosphere of the demoralized districts of New York. Although much of the local housing is squalid beyond belief, the homeless population is small and the dispossessed stratum so conspicuous in most Latin American capitals is absent (Caplow et al. 1964:224).

In San Juan, Caplow, Stryker and Wallace concluded, satisfaction prevails with "housing, neighborhood, amenities, public services, and the entire urban environment." And they agreed with the findings of Tumin and Feldman that "there is very high morale in all segments of the Puerto Rican community . . . members of all classes feel well integrated" (1961:164).

According to Oscar Lewis, however, these conclusions are "rather broad and overly optimistic" and "in sharp contrast" with his findings about slum families in San Juan (1965:xiv). Gordon Lewis (1963:15) cited the Tumin and Feldman study as an example of the characteristic defects of the American sociological imagination and literature. And in their study of schizophrenia among slum families in San Juan, Rogler and Hollingshead found a marked lack of integration in both shantytown and housing project.

Beyond the extended family, the neighborhood is not integrated on a cooperative basis; rather, relations with neighbors are conflict ridden. Almost all husbands and wives are quick to recite a history of accumulated grievances against the neighbors who are derogated as dirty, noisy, immoral and inconsiderate (1964:408).

In fact, the rural migrant in San Juan longs intensely for a home in the suburbs which is large enough for his family, has healthy living conditions, and provides the privacy which permits friendly and respectful relations with neighbors.

Stresses of the Migrants in San Juan

In view of the intense stress on the people in the culture of poverty in Puerto Rico, it is not surprising to find that schizophrenia and other forms of psychopathology are concentrated unduly among persons of low socioeconomic status. According to Rogler and Hollingshead, schizophrenia was the mental illness found most frequently among 1,500 patients at the public mental health hospital in San Juan. Based on an estimate of at least 10,000 schizophrenics who were living with their families, "a rate of 435 psychotics per 100,000 population" was indicated for Puerto Rico as a whole (Fitzpatrick and Gould 1968:31). Very many of the slum families described by Oscar Lewis in *La Vida* had "a history of psychopathology which goes back a few generations," and which includes "epileptic-type hysterical seizures, commonly known as the 'Puerto Rican syndrome' " (1965:xxviii–xxix).

In their study, Rogler and Hollingshead attempted to discover whether, among the very poor, "the lives of persons who develop schizophrenia differ from those of persons who are not schizophrenics." They found no significant differences between the two groups (1964:401). Their sample population consisted of almost 5,500 people in about 1,100 households, with every household in the San Juan metropolitan area having an equal probability of being chosen. This population was stratified into five classes on the basis of occupation and education, and two out of three persons in San Juan were found to be in Class V. From the sample population, two groups of Class V persons, each consisting of twenty families, were selected and studied intensively. In the experimental group, either the husband or the wife in each family was schizophrenic, or both were. In the control group of nonschizophrenic families, the subjects were neurotic, had personality disorders, or had no symptoms. The forty families represented a population in which the parents were between twenty and thirty-nine years old and had never been treated for mental illness. About 65 percent of the families lived in slums, the rest in housing projects. The mean number of people per household was 5.8.

Three generations were studied: the subjects, their families of orientation, and their families of procreation. The families of orientation of both groups were found to be similar socially and culturally; thus there was no relationship between their mental status and their economic level, education, composition, and stability.

No correlation was found between migration and mental illness, since five out of six people in the study were rural migrants. "Mental illness is ascribed to some member of one-half of the families of orientation" (Rogler and Hollingshead 1964:404), although schizophrenia in the subjects was not linked to mental illness in their families of orientation.

More than half the parents of the subjects completed less than a year of school, and the fathers were predominantly farm laborers. About 95 percent of the subjects suffered economic hardship in childhood, and all left school because of pressing economic problems. Serious family problems were the rule, due largely to the adulterous and drunken behavior of fathers. Half of the families of orientation were broken by the death or desertion of one or more of the parents, usually the father, and the children were distributed among relatives. More often the subjects preferred their mothers to their fathers.

The socioeconomic difficulties of the subjects were continuously exacerbated by the increasing incongruity of traditional cultural roles in an industrialized urban setting. When the conflicts proved too onerous and an individual could no longer function in the traditional roles, or when one more stress was added to an already heavy burden, mental breakdown resulted. "The culture and their low socioeconomic status in the society present them with a series of tension points that are linked to the difficulties they have faced through the years" (Rogler and Hollingshead 1964:405).

The major tension points arise from unemployment; insufficient income; the death of a child; traditional cultural values about the roles of men and women; the cultural horror of psychopathology. A very deep source of strain is the gap between aspirations and achievement. The agricultural worker's desire for upward mobility, the basic reason for migration to the city, is intensified by exposure to the affluence of the upper classes and of tourists in San Juan. "The elegant parapets of the San Juan tourist palaces almost overlook the fetid slums of the San Juan city districts. Income inequality is reinforced" (G. Lewis 1963: 312–13). The communications media constantly advertise products as status symbols, and the migrants buy on credit furniture and appliances which are repossessed when payments cannot be met. "Usually these families do not know the extent of their debts and efforts are made to meet only the most immediate and pressing expenses" (Rogler and Hollingshead 1964:285). "Widespread recourse to credit and indebtedness becomes . . . the index of widespread status panic. It seems at

times as if the society is nothing much more than a culture of anxiety"
(G. Lewis 1963:257).

The schizophrenic families lived much the same way as the well families until about five years before the onset of the disorder, when either
economic problems or physical illness increased sharply, which could
have occurred as well among the control families as among the experimental families. "At a recent and discernible period in the life arc
prior to the eruption of overt symptomatology, a rash of insoluble,
mutually reenforcing problems emerge to trap the persons" (Rogler and
Hollingshead 1964:413).

About 73 percent of the husbands had full-time jobs; 12 percent
worked part time, and the remainder were unemployed. The sick and
well men started to work at about the same age, had the same number
of jobs for about the same length of time, and were unemployed to
about the same extent. However, the mean monthly income of the sick
men for all their jobs was about $87, while for the well men it was
about $115 (Rogler and Hollingshead 1964:289). The sick men asso-
ciated the beginning of their illness with an abrupt drop in earnings,
which resulted from unemployment, or increasing job absences, or an
inability to obtain normal salary increases.

With the onset of schizophrenia the problems of the sick men in
their jobs "are more dramatic, more profound, and more agonizing
than those of the well men."

The sick man becomes a ready scapegoat for his associates and bosses. He
is too anxious, too doubt ridden, too inept in the verbal repartee which is
an admired skill among his associates to have anything more than peripheral
membership in his work group (Rogler and Hollingshead 1964:290).

The role reversals that take place when the men and women in the
culture of poverty succumb to schizophrenia seem to demonstrate that
they find the traditional roles dysfunctional and onerous, for they reject
them when they are no longer bound by the usual constraints.

The economic difficulties that ensue when the husband is ill lead to
quarrels only when the wife is also ill. Whether or not the husband is
ill, the schizophrenic wife complains bitterly about insufficient financial
support. But the typical wife does not blame her husband for inadequate
support for she knows that jobs are few, irregular, and low paying.
Most of the well women want very much to work in order to improve
the family's standard of living. But the husband who is not ill prevents
his wife from working because he fears "the general trend toward the
greater freedom of women which has accompanied the increasing urbanization, industrialization and Americanization of Puerto Rico" (O. Lewis

1965:xxvii). However, about half the women who are married to schizophrenic men work outside the home, because soon after the men become ill they can no longer earn a living. "Neither the control families nor the families in which only the wife is sick experience the problem of economic survival as acutely and as dramatically as do the families with sick men" (Rogler and Hollingshead 1964:302).

As the working and social worlds gradually withdraw from the sick man, his home becomes his only haven. His wife considers this an increment, for in the well families the husband is rarely at home and the wife is always there. When the wife works, the schizophrenic husband learns to take care of the house, but he is very suspicious of her outside activities. The wife realizes that the role reversal is very threatening, and in marked contrast to the typical husband's attitude toward the money he earns, she gives her husband all her earnings so that he may continue to dispense the funds.

Under the double sex standard marital fidelity is violated far more by the husband, in his role of *macho,* than by the wife. "The percentage of husbands in the present generation who have been involved in adulterous behavior is almost the same as it was in the parental generation." Since sex is considered essential to the man, the wife very soon learns to use sex to manipulate and control her husband. When the husband is mentally ill, the wife is generally compliant sexually, particularly since he is now less demanding. But when the wife is schizophrenic, she completely rebels against her traditional sexual role and repeatedly rejects her husband's advances. When both husband and wife are ill, "sexual intercourse is employed by each spouse to humiliate and degrade the other" (Rogler and Hollingshead 1964:333–334, 346).

Generally the families in which the husband is ill are very harmonious. The sick man is defenseless, at the opposite pole from the dominant male in the typical family. "The union in husband-schizophrenic families resembles a . . . relationship between an emotionally supportive, martyrlike but controlling mother and a tyrannical but dependent son" (Rogler and Hollingshead 1964:307). The pattern of *respeto* between husband and wife is much less strictly enforced, for they are united in the common quest for solutions to the problems created by his illness, and the wife guides him to all the therapeutic sources—druggists, psychiatrists, *curanderas,* Spiritualists.

Psychotic breaks from reality which involve aggressive and uncoordinated outbursts against other persons are seldom experienced by the sick men who also rarely exhibit the trancelike episodes of going berserk, as do sick women (Rogler and Hollingshead 1964:312).

But the sick wife violates the *respeto* relationship. She openly resents her husband's freedom and privileges, and engages him in a struggle for power. But she is very much afraid of him. "Her fear of his rough commands often borders on panic, as evidenced by her trembling and stuttering when her husband comes home." The husband has no insight into his wife's illness.

He seldom, if ever entertains the possibility that his own behavior seriously harms his wife . . . even though she often tells him that his excessive rectitude, his authoritarian comportment and the severe beatings he inflicts are making her illness worse (Rogler and Hollingshead 1964:318–319).

The mother frequently becomes schizophrenic after the death of a child. The death of ten out of twelve children in seven families was followed by the onset of schizophrenia in the mother. The mother in the one family in the control group which suffered such a death exhibited very neurotic symptoms. When the mother is schizophrenic she cannot give the children the emotional support they receive from the well mother, and the family becomes disorganized. The "significant association between a schizophrenic mother and severely disturbed behavior in the children" (Rogler and Hollingshead 1964:400) is usually reflected in scholastic retardation.

The harmonious families of the sick men are in striking contrast. "Their children are the least retarded in school and none of these families has severe behavioral problems among the children" (Rogler and Hollingshead 1964:399). In the average family the wife protects the children against the father's excessive physical punishment, but this is seldom necessary when the father is ill:

the sick men married to well women . . . more than men in any other diagnostic group, spend many hours with the children. . . . Even though the sick men are subject to erratic moments of explosive outbursts, they are, on the whole, benevolent, gentle, and emotionally committed fathers (Rogler and Hollingshead 1964:384).

More than 90 percent of the families in the study had relatives living in the San Juan area, with whom the well families were involved in a network of mutual aid. But when the wife becomes ill, the relationships of both spouses with the relatives are seriously affected. The husband projects on his wife's family the hostility or indifference he feels for his wife, and "schizophrenic women . . . are engaged in an incessant war against their in-laws, particularly their mother-in-law" (Rogler and Hollingshead 1964:375). When the husband is ill, the wife's kinfolk rally to her financial and emotional support, but the abnormal involvement of the wife's relatives leads to isolation from the husband's kin and to a loss of autonomy and privacy for the family. This becomes another source of tension for the husband.

The marital conflicts, the disruption of the nuclear and extended families, the adverse effects on the children when the wife is schizophrenic all "serve to reaffirm the functional importance of the woman's role in preserving the inner coherence of the family." The husband might be more tolerant if the wife had a visible physical handicap instead of mental illness, but even then it is unlikely that he would "assume a supportive role and perform all the functions associated with the women's role." It is "difficult, if not impossible," for the husband to "perform role functions inconsistent with the norms of masculinity which pervade the culture and according to which the men are socialized" (Rogler and Hollingshead 1964:418).

The woman's ability to cope with her husband's illness also derives from her traditional role. Women learn at an early age to provide emotional and therapeutic support, not only in the nuclear and extended families, but also in their cultural roles as midwife, *curandera,* and Spiritualist medium. But when a wife must cope with her husband's illness and with child rearing and also provide economic support for the family, her health is usually severely impaired. The women with the schizophrenic husbands have a rate of physical illness that is "almost four times that of the women in the control group" (Rogler and Hollingshead 1964:417).

The role reversals that take place among men and women who are schizophrenic indicate that the longings of each sex for more flexible roles, which are normally suppressed, burst forth when mental illness demolishes the cultural constraints. Or perhaps the inability to play the prescribed roles when stress is very great results in schizophrenia. The schizophrenic men become dependent, supportive, benevolent, and gentle, and the schizophrenic women become aggressive and combative in their desperate reach for equality. Each sex seems to take on the major role traits assigned to the other, so that the families in which the men are ill become harmonious because both husband and wife play the "feminine" nurturant role, but the families in which the wife is ill become arenas of power struggles because both spouses play the "masculine" role of aggression and competition. "What we consider 'madness'—whether it appears in women or men is either (a) the acting out of the female experience or (b) the rejection of one's sex-role stereotype" (Chesler 1971:271).

A very severe problem confronting the lower-class schizophrenic in

Puerto Rico is the cultural condemnation of *locura*. Even professional people are fearful and fatalistic about mental illness, and in all classes the family attempts to keep secret the mental illness of one of its members. But in the slums and housing projects, schizophrenics generally live with their families, and they cannot conceal their deviant behavior from their neighbors, who torment them.

People mock them, throw stones at them and provoke them to see them react in as bizarre a way as possible. . . . The person who becomes mentally ill . . . is nicknamed "loco," and very often his real name is not used in referring to him. As far as employment opportunities are concerned, there are practically none (Martínez 1957:64).

Outside of the family, the schizophrenic has only one source of acceptance and support, the Spiritualist medium. In four-fifths of the families in the study at least one spouse was a Spiritualist; in almost half the families both spouses were Spiritualists. Even though it is opposed by both branches of Christianity, two-thirds of the Catholics and one-half of the Protestants in Puerto Rico believe in Spiritualism, and the belief is particularly widespread in the lower classes. The Spiritualist medium, like the revivalist pastor, understands the poor because she is herself a member of their subculture. She provides social support and prestige for the emotionally disturbed person by representing him as endowed with *facultades*. Spiritualist sessions are similar in some ways to group psychotherapy, and are "institutionalized to discharge the tensions and anxieties generated in other areas of social life." Thus Spiritualism is a form of "folk psychiatry, serving its believers without their paying the penalty of community stigma associated with psychiatric agencies." In fact, for the majority of migrants in San Juan, "outside the nuclear and extended family, religious beliefs and practices are the most important source of social support" (Rogler and Hollingshead 1964:248, 254, 259).

Mitigation of Stresses

The rural migrants in Puerto Rico are faced not only with severe stresses and problems, but also with the advantages deriving from the great progress in education and health that took place between 1940 and 1965. In this period illiteracy decreased by almost two-thirds, dropping from 32 percent to 11 percent (O. Lewis 1965:xiv). Malaria was wiped out, and the death rate was enormously reduced. Deaths from diarrhea and enteritis decreased from 405 per 100,000 to 39;

tuberculosis, from 260 to 17; pneumonia, from 169 to 30. Infant mortality decreased from 113 to 44 per 100,000, and general mortality, from about 20 to about 7 per 100,000.[3] The suicide rate also declined by about two-thirds, from 30.7 in 1936 to 9.7 per 100,000 in 1960 (Senior 1961:82), which was about the same rate as in the United States.

The decline by about two-thirds in illiteracy, the general mortality rate, and the suicide rate, all in approximately the same period, illuminates the relationships among education, economics, and physical and mental health. This decline clearly demonstrates that many fewer people are now in the culture of poverty than 30 years ago. Oscar Lewis's claim that the culture of poverty tends to be self-perpetuating because of its early effects on the children would apply more to a static society with a stagnating economy than to a country like Puerto Rico, where many children of rural migrants do take advantage of new opportunities. Those who are still in the culture of poverty, however, perhaps two-thirds of the rural migrants in San Juan, are living under extremely stressful circumstances because of continuing social and economic problems, poor physical and mental health, and dysfunctional sex roles.

---

[3]Commonwealth of Puerto Rico, *A Summary in Facts & Figures,* p. 4.

PART III

UNITED STATES:
CULTURAL-HISTORICAL PERSPECTIVE

CHAPTER 8

The American Heritage

> Though sectional, economic and religious differences are highly significant in some respects, there are certain themes that transcend these variations. Some life goals, some basic attitudes tend to be shared by Americans of every region and of all social classes (C. Kluckhohn 1965:197).

The themes, life goals, and attitudes shared by Americans are rooted in the influences stemming from Puritanism and the frontier experience, and from the relationships between the descendants of the original settlers and the other peoples of the United States.

The themes that emerged in the course of the historical development of the nation gave rise to counterthemes. The quest for material wealth was accompanied by a sense of mission; individual responsibility, by the longing for community; competitiveness, by voluntary cooperation; conformity to law and order, by resistance to authority; risk-taking, by the yearning for security; ceaseless activity and restlessness, by the desire for surcease; confidence in the mastery over nature, by the search for nostrums; worship of success, by belief in the worth of the common man; optimism about the future, by widespread anxiety.

The most damaging strains on the national equilibrium arose from the dichotomy between the great emphasis upon equality and the condition of inequality imposed upon the Indians, the blacks, and the later immigrants.

The Europeans Who Became Americans

The historical events leading to the European settlement of the New World constitute a basic source of the values, for immigration was the experience common to all. The immigrants shared certain cultural patterns and characteristics. The vast majority were displaced persons who came from Europe, a culture area where a relatively high premium was placed on personal achievement. Among the hordes of the dispossessed in Europe, the immigrants were those who made the decision to leave, and the people who reached the New World, particularly in the early period, were those who survived the dangerous and difficult crossing. Thus, the immigrants were generally uprooted people, with individual initiative, the ability to survive, and the goal of personal achievement.

The breakdown of medieval Europe displaced masses of people, and the Americas provided the solution they were desperately seeking. In seventeenth-century England, the concentration of land into great estates drove thousands of peasants to the villages and towns, and the excess labor destroyed the traditional bargaining power of the skilled worker. Thus the dislocation of the peasant displaced the artisan, and there was no place for either in the changing society, except London. Between 1550 and 1660 the population of London increased from about 90,000 to some 500,000, and the "sturdy vagabonds" lived "heaped up together and in a sort smothered, with many families . . . in one . . . small tenement; and yet, still others continued to arrive" (Handlin 1963:19).

With no way of making a living in England, many of the dispossessed were drawn to the colonies, where the unlimited land was cheap or free, and there was a crying need for labor. Indentured servitude paid for the passage of the majority who had no resources. But indentured servants did not satisfy the demand for labor, and involuntary labor was recruited from three sources: Irish war prisoners in the 1640s; English and Scottish debtors, paupers, and criminals; slaves from West Africa, especially after 1660. When they arrived in the New World, the British were sold as servants, with the prospect of future freedom, but for the blacks, the period of servitude was unlimited.

The same processes of socioeconomic breakdown and propulsion of emigrants across the Atlantic took place in one European country after another until well into the twentieth century. For more than a thousand years European society was relatively stable. The backbone and bulk of this society were the peasants who lived in villages dominated by the lord and the Church, and integrated by ties of family, the functional social and economic unit.

For the lord's protection against hostile outsiders and for the spiritual ministrations of the Church, the peasant paid in labor, rents, and tithes, and since his holding was small, he could never accumulate a reserve against natural and man-made catastrophes. Although he rebelled from time to time when the lord was unusually capricious or the burdens became intolerable, generally the peasant accepted his lot. Poverty sapped his spirit, and fatalism helped him endure.

The population in Europe had remained stable for centuries, but in the seventeenth century, infant mortality began to decline. Between 1750 and 1850 the population almost doubled (Handlin 1952:25), and it increased at an even faster rate after that. The peasant had to subdivide his small plot among his more numerous sons, and all became even poorer, subsisting mainly on the potato, which had been brought in from the New World.

In order to obtain enough cash to hold on to the land, men began to sell their labor seasonally outside of their villages, then farther and farther away, until finally they were migrating periodically to foreign countries. Thus arose a new social class of migratory workers. Some drifted into the cities, which were expanding with the growth of commerce and industry. The larger urban population augmented demands on agricultural production, and landowners, especially in England and the Netherlands, began to use scientific techniques to increase crops and cattle. But only large land concentrations could be exploited scientifically and, supported by the merchants who profited from greater production of grain and wool, land enclosure accelerated. The peasants, now forced to raise crops for the market, could not compete with the large landowners. The number of the destitute mounted as agriculture expanded, crops failed, and famine and epidemics raged.

With starvation the only alternative, more and more peasants took the arduous journey across the Atlantic, followed by artisans, mill operatives, miners, and factory workers. Ethnic enclaves in America drew relatives and friends in a mighty procession, and in less than a century and a half, more than 35 million people came to the New World.

In this common flow were gathered up people of the most diverse qualities, people whose rulers had for centuries been enemies, people who had not even known of each other's existence. Now they would share each other's future (Handlin 1952:35).

They came from the British Isles, from Germany and Scandinavia, from south, east, and central Europe, and from Asia Minor. "It was immensely significant that the first step to the New World, despite all the hazards it involved, was the outcome of a desperate individual choice" (Handlin 1952:38). The immigrants to America opted for "Change, Chance, Choice," which forced them to create a new way of life, a new philosophy, and new kinds of energy.

They chose change, to actively transplant old roots, and then were forced to find new roots in Change itself. They took a chance and then had to revere Chance. . . . They created a new elite out of the types of men who fit this new world (Erikson 1964:84).

Most of the men who made their way to North America were humble in origin and had little formal learning. The handful of doctors, lawyers, ministers, and younger sons of the gentry were generally persons who had failed, or who could find no outlet at home for their ambition and restlessness. Only a few came solely for adventure or gold. A small minority were religious and political refugees with exceptional skills and important commercial and intellectual connections. Those who came during most of the nineteenth century "could not impose their own ways upon society; but neither were they constrained to conform to those already established" (Handlin 1952:5). They had the space and the opportunity to seek land and wealth, to set up private utopias, and to try again if they failed.

Europeans became Americans because they no sooner arrived than they immediately felt the effects of plenty. Their toils were no less heavy than before but . . . they had put behind them involuntary idleness, servile dependence, penury and useless labor. . . . They became landowners. . . . *They ceased to be ciphers and felt themselves men because they were treated as such.* They were then Americans (Handlin 1963:77).

The Influence of Puritanism

The term "Puritanism" denotes the theological, ethical, social, and political philosophy and way of life typical of certain Protestant groups that arose in "a European civilization, which had always, in contrast with other world cultures, placed a particularly high premium on personal achievement." The development of Puritanism near the end of the 16th century reflected the increasing importance of the goal of individual economic achievement: ". . . it was to be the special genius of Englishmen, from Elizabeth's time onward, to transform this career concept from its earlier chivalric form into one of economic fulfillment —from 'glory' to 'success' " (Elkins 1959:43).

Puritanism rested on the Calvinist concept of predestination, the bestowal of grace at birth upon the elect. The sign of selection to grace was success in professional activity. This was the reward for worldly asceticism, a type of rigorous self-control in all areas of life, exercised to glorify and obey God. The word of God was understood not through the mediation of another person, but only by the individual mind. Thus each person was responsible for his relationship with God and the salvation of his soul. The virtues which were extolled as most pleasing to God—sobriety, prudence, diligence, thrift, and moderation—were proving to be those which led also to commercial success.

These values not only contributed to the expansion of business, but also played an important part in changing traditional attitudes toward social obligations. For 150 years the British Crown and Church, acting on the principle that ownership of land and wealth carried duties as well as privileges, had protected "peasants against landlords, craftsmen against merchants, and consumers against middlemen" (Tawney 1958: 272). But when the rights of property came to be accepted as primary, enclosure was legalized, the peasants were driven off the land, and buyers were protected only by the "natural" laws of supply and demand. The concept of the social character of wealth increasingly lost ground to the view that help to the poor fostered improvidence and idleness and was counter to God's will. As success in business was "at once the sign and reward of ethical superiority" (Tawney 1958:270), so failure became proof of vice or personal inadequacy.

The Puritans viewed the possession of great wealth as dangerous only because it might lead to idleness and self-indulgence. The safest and most rewarding form of activity was in a calling, which ensured rational conduct, regular habits, and protected rich and poor alike against the temptations of the flesh. Time that was not spent in work, in the calling, was time wasted, and wasting time was a deadly sin. The emphasis upon each man's need for a calling led later to Adam Smith's apotheosis of the division of labor (Weber 1960:569).

The Puritans became "particularly adept in organizing undertakings and . . . in rationalizing economic action." While the Puritan ethic did not create capitalism, it certainly contributed to the development of the spirit of capitalism.

Puritanism in its later phases added a halo of ethical sanctification to the appeal of economic expediency, and offered a moral creed, in which the duties of religion and the calls of business ended their long estrangement in unanticipated reconciliation (Tawney 1958:272).

In the Protestant countries, the Puritan ethic led to the positive social valuation of the pursuit of science as a calling. Empiricism and rationalism were implicit in the Puritan value of success in worldly matters, and it was the joining of empiricism to rationalism that distinguished modern science. It was not only for the glory of God but also for the benefit of mankind that the Puritan scientists investigated the secrets of nature, combining spiritual and material pursuits in a typically Puritan framework. Contrary to Tawney's view that the Puritans did not acknowledge social responsibility, Merton states that "the second dominant tenet in the Puritan ethos designated social welfare, the good of the many, as a goal ever to be held in mind" (Merton 1959:332).

As a philosophy, Puritanism made a tremendous contribution to political freedom and the concept of individualism.

The foundation of democracy is the sense of spiritual independence which nerves the individual to stand alone against the power of this world. . . . The virtues of enterprise, diligence and thrift are the indispensable foundation of any complex and vigorous civilization (Tawney 1958:286).

In the New World the Puritans planted the seeds of what was to become the American business civilization. Not only did they derive principally from the commercial and financial classes, but they crossed the Atlantic, backed by corporations, to profit from trade. However, they left behind comfortable homes and social positions to endure the rigors of the wilderness because they were also "antiestablishment" individualists, religious dissidents with a sense of mission, convinced they had been chosen to establish a new way of life that would be a model for all people everywhere. "For we must consider that we shall be as a city upon a hill, the eyes of all people are upon us" (Winthrop 1961:34). This sense of mission became a most important part of the American heritage.

The Puritan population of New England increased rapidly and formed a society which governed itself. "They continually exercised the rights of sovereignty; they named their magistrates, concluded peace or declared war, made police regulations and enacted laws, as if their allegiance was due only to God" (Tocqueville 1956:43). By 1650 they had established townships and were keeping public records of every kind. They taxed themselves to provide for the poor and to establish and maintain compulsory education so that every child might learn to read the Bible.

But the Puritan governments in Massachusetts and Connecticut became theocratic, "merciless alike to religious liberty and economic license" (Tawney 1958:271). The legislators were mainly concerned with the maintenance of moral and orderly behavior, which they enforced by unsparing punishment of infractions. Church attendance was compulsory, and "conformity and exile were the only alternatives to mutilation, branding and scourging." Puritan women were rigidly restricted. The religious hysteria of the witch hunts centered on women, and "Quaker women were flogged from town to town" (Martindale 1960:282).

But disaffected Puritans, Quakers, and other nonconformists found a haven in Rhode Island and Pennsylvania. These states, "whose tolerant, individualist and utilitarian temper was destined to find the greatest representative in the golden common sense of Benjamin Franklin" (Tawney 1958:271), undermined the Puritan theocracies. Thus, in the wide spaces of America the values of conformity and nonconformity, both deriving from Puritanism, had room to flourish and to play their part in the development of the national character.

The heritage which the English Puritans left to their American descendants included the values of individual responsibility and initiative; thrift, diligence, and sobriety; work as an end in itself, and ceaseless activity; success as a reward for striving, and failure as a measure of personal inadequacy; orientation to the future; utilitarianism, rationalism, empiricism, and pragmatism; respect for science; a sense of mission; conformity, and resistance to authority.

New England supplied a large proportion of the pioneers, who carried the Puritan traditions to the frontier, where they duplicated the patterns of the original English settlers.

Many of these men, who rush so boldly onwards in pursuit of wealth, were already in the enjoyment of a competency in their own part of the country. They take their wives along with them and make them share the countless perils and privations that always attend the commencement of these expeditions (Tocqueville 1956:237).

The Influence of the Frontier

The frontier has been a predominant influence in the shaping of American character and culture, in the molding of American political life and institutions (C. Kluckhohn 1965:209).

From the time of the first Pilgrim settlement in 1620 to the end of the nineteenth century, the settlement of the nation was "the most important common experience in North America" (Martindale 1960:240). The frontier, according to Frederick Jackson Turner, fostered democracy, nationalism, and individualism. It was the true melting pot, where pioneers from every region and from many countries endured common rigors. The basis of Jacksonian democracy was "the good fellowship and genuine social feeling of the frontier in which classes and inequalities of fortune played little part" (Turner 1920:302). New democratic movements began in the West, "including more general suffrage, free schools, state education and easier qualifications for political office" (Martindale 1960:243).

By the early nineteenth century, the frontier had greatly weakened the traditional patriarchal family. Sons who could establish themselves on their own land early in life had little regard for filial obedience and subordination. Pioneer women carried their full share of the burdens and hardships, and achieved practical equality with men, for the brutal frontier conditions "established a certain rough egalitarianism which challenged other, long-established concepts of propriety." In 1889, when the Wyoming legislators found that they could enter the Union only by abandoning woman's suffrage, they said: "We will remain out of the Union a hundred years rather than come in without the women" (Flexner 1959:9, 178).

The frontier promoted nationalism and a sense of nationality in the American people. It stimulated legislation, especially in the territories, which developed the power of the federal government and militated against sectionalism. And during the nineteenth century, the mythology of the frontier formed the basis for a national American literature. Above all, the influence of the frontier reinforced the Puritan value of individualism, which was at the heart of the whole American movement.

Summing up the qualities which the national character owed to the frontier, Turner wrote:

That coarseness and strength combined with acuteness and inquisitiveness; that practical, inventive turn of mind, quick to find expedients; that masterful grasp of material things, lacking in the artistic but powerful to effect great ends; that restless, nervous energy; that dominant individualism, working for good and for evil, and withal that buoyancy and exuberance which comes with freedom—these are the traits of the frontier, or traits called out elsewhere because of the existence of the frontier (Turner 1920:37).

The patterns established by the first pioneers were continued by successive generations. The trail was blazed by the fur trappers and traders, men who could live with the Indians and the animals of the forest. Then came the pioneer families, who subsisted by hunting and fishing while they fought off the Indians and cleared the land. Finally the "agents of civilization" arrived—the land speculators, lawyers, officials, shopkeepers and artisans. And the pioneers, faced with the choice of settling down to farming or selling their claims and moving on, generally continued westward, "disqualified by temperament and character from adjusting to a routine" (Handlin 1963:204).

Founded mainly by trading companies, the new settlements turned to commerce even as they were trying to gain a toehold in the wilderness. From the beginning, fur trapping, fishing, and agriculture were shaped to develop in a money market, and capitalism emerged "as the principal dynamic force in American society" (Elkins 1959:43).

The essence of business was speculation. Everyone with a surplus of capital vied for the government grants of land and speculated in land. Although the merchants and larger landowners obtained the greatest benefits through their political connections, the smaller man also made money. Artisans and professional people were in great demand, were well paid, and could accumulate money for speculation. Farmers specialized in crops that would bring good prices at the market, supplemented their income by fishing and the manufacture of articles from farm products, made loans, opened stores, and speculated in land. Many farmers acquired great estates and were limited only by the shortage of labor.

"Everyone who could afford it was greedy for a share of the future that each advance into the wilderness revealed" (Handlin 1963:89). Each man succeeded or failed on his own, and those who failed tried again or became subsistence farmers. Fortunes were never secure because money was always being invested in new undertakings.

A situation that compelled men who cherished security constantly to seek out and to take risks formed the character of the Americans. . . . Ceaseless striving and mobility were necessary to hold on, for only expansion could preserve what had already been created (Handlin 1963:155).

The early proprietors tried to institute feudal socioeconomic patterns. But the men who had pulled up their roots and endured the hazardous crossing rejected servile dependency on a landlord; "it was too easy even for the poor who were free to remain their own masters" (Handlin 1963:95). The crying need for labor dictated just and decent treatment of servants. Even in New England controls weakened in the wake of a population that dispersed at will, that could leave for other colonies offering more freedom. "Masters and artisans were ever less responsive to . . . conscience in setting prices." New families that were successful elbowed those that had established themselves earlier. "Shifts in status came quickly and easily and mobility emptied the formal rankings of significance" (Handlin 1963:36).

Wherever they settled, the colonists needed local government and laws to ensure the orderly conduct of their affairs. "The wilderness, once men learned to exploit it, offered them all the goods their hearts desired; it most lacked regularity, predictability, security." Everywhere political power developed in a direction opposite to that in Europe. Instead of passing downward from the throne, "authority accumulated on the local level and passed upward by the representation of those who held it" (Handlin 1963:54, 49). The governor had to deal with men who held power in the towns and counties, and local officeholders had to consider the interests of the communities if they were to survive and grow. Men accepted rule by the powerful and wealthy as the price for order, but the assent of the ruled was established early as a political principle, for they felt obliged to obey only when their rights were protected by their rulers.

Since neither law books nor lawyers were always available, laws had to be improvised in response to specific situations. The lawmakers referred to the Bible and to learned texts, the teachings of the ministers, and particularly to experience. Although these men were motivated by self-interest, "they were also guided by some notion of what was just; religious faith and habit persuaded them that there was a standard by which to recognize and punish wrongs, by which to resolve disputes and by which to preserve the peace." But the colonists also learned that laws were not sacred and could be changed. Since exact records were kept and precedents compiled only in New England, each man had to be vigilant to protect his own interests. "Hence the sensitivity of the colonists to their liberties, which meant privileges or rights" (Handlin 1963:55, 56).

Quite early in the history of the colonies the lower classes began to question orders instead of accepting them unthinkingly. There was "a weakening of the habit of deference to the great ones of the land, a disposition to talk back" (Handlin 1963:111). By the middle of the eighteenth century, farmers, artisans, and religious dissenters were not only voting but also putting up their own candidates. In fact, the assurance of extensive rights for all helped to draw new settlers to the colonies.

According to Turner, the frontier released the individual from complex European institutions into the primitive simplicity of the wilderness, where he emerged as a self-reliant, self-sufficient man. The regression that occurred as civilized standards were lowered was equated by Turner (1920) with the "primitive" life of the Indian. Handlin (1963), however, views the regression as the result of the decline of communal controls which accompanied the physical isolation of each family. Without these controls, "rural life everywhere in the colonies grew increasingly disorderly" (1963:100). Men went their own way, neither interfering with anyone else, nor brooking interference. In many regions the inn was the meeting place, and the holding of court was marked by violence and drunkenness which erupted from "pent-up conviviality."

In their loneliness, boredom, fear, and physical discomfort, people drank huge amounts of liquor.

"For all, the days passed in a grim round, scarcely marked by feast or ceremony," according to Handlin. Literacy declined, and "the curse . . . entered common speech." The behavior of the children reflected the increasingly rude manners of the parents. "Children and servants were disobedient, and husband and wife abused one another" (1963: 101, 102). Sons could hardly wait until they were old enough to strike out on their own, and after years of hardship and striving, parents found themselves alone in the promised land.

Courtship lost its traditional restraints, even in New England. It became customary for couples to spend evenings together in bed, presumably to economize on light and heat. Before the end of the seventeenth century, marriage had become secularized in many parts of North America, and the family became "an arrangement . . . in which two individuals undertook to work together for the satisfaction of their own ends" (Handlin 1963:41).

The frontier produced "men and women who learned to live without restraints imposed from without or inherited from the past. . . . Few were able to satisfy the urges that pressed them on in search for more" (Handlin 1963:102). In the wilderness Americans obtained riches from the soil, but they became increasingly uncertain of all other goals.

Before the end of the seventeenth century the second and third generations predominated in the affairs of the colonies. They were more at home in the wilderness than their immigrant parents had ever been and were confident they could conquer it.

They were rootless, mobile and unstable; but . . . they were . . . not subject to the strains of the decision that had burdened their parents or grandparents. They were likely to accept as a way of life . . . the disorder and precariousness that troubled the immigrants (Handlin 1963:70).

During the first century and a half, even in New England, the colonies became increasingly secular. People learned to accept each other as individuals instead of members of a religious group. Dissenters were among the most respected men, and the minister ceased to be the spokesman for the community. But the decline of established religion affected education profoundly. The seventeenth-century schools had been primarily religious, and they now seemed irrelevant to practical matters, especially in the rural areas. Children were taught to read, write and "reckon," but elementary education stagnated until the nineteenth century. However, informal education continued through the new media, newspapers and magazines, which increasingly became the most important sources of information and the molders of public opinion. Scholars addressed the people directly and through the press, and learning was not a function of status.

About the middle of the eighteenth century, religion revived with the Great Awakening. It was a new kind of religion, a religion of repentance and redemption, preached by offshoots of the established churches. Those who had forsaken the faith of their fathers could now save themselves from damnation by ethical behavior. Conscience and reason now became the only guides to action, and since all could share in the hope of salvation, "there was some common element of worth in every man, whatever his place, rank or station" (Handlin 1963:128). Thus Puritanism, based on the salvation of an elite, was democratized, reflecting the social and political democratization that was taking place.

Revivalism drew the settlers together, mainly on a nonsectarian basis, for the purpose of improving society. They established new schools and colleges and tried to improve conditions in the cities. They helped the poor, the sick, the aged, and the slaves, and attempted to moderate the use of liquor. People began to talk about a just form of government that would enable all to lead the good life:

the Great Awakening was a component in the success of the American Revolution, for it promoted a common consciousness among Americans from Virginia to Massachusetts . . . "sweeping away old traditions, stimulating independence and enthusiasm" (Martindale 1960:283).

The major political and social changes that had been taking place for a century were legitimized by the Revolution, which was successfully concluded because of "an organizational genius for self-government acquired over generations" (Elkins 1959:146). The Revolutionary War, fought for the rights of common men, encouraged these men to assert themselves after the war ended.

Called on to protest, to fight in the armies and to show concern for the rights of man, they became active participants in government, citizens rather than subjects; and they showed no disposition to sink back to an inferior position when the crisis was over (Handlin 1963:174).

The struggle for independence, the terms used to justify it, and the provisions of the Constitution and the Bill of Rights "prevented the United States from subjugating other peoples . . . and required . . . that it adopt a sympathetic view of the struggles of other men for liberty" (Handlin 1963:144). As the pioneers swept across the continent, extending the borders of the country, altruistic ideals and the hope of gain were meshed inextricably together.

But the ideals had at least this influence, that neither in thought nor in action did it occur to Americans to make subjects of the people of the territories added to the Union. All were to be Americans, citizens of states absolutely equal in rights with those of 1776 (Handlin 1963:208).

After the Revolution, political leaders in the new frontier states came increasingly from the lower classes. At the same time signs of social strain began to appear in various parts of the country, particularly along the frontier. Thousands of farmers turned away from the dominant values of the nation, "gave up the struggle for individuality and achievement . . . abjured private property," and joined the Shakers and similar movements. In the 1790s and thereafter, revivalism swept regularly through the frontier, feeding "on the pent-up tensions of people constantly forced by their struggles to doubt their own adequacy" (Handlin 1963:128, 191). Although they were conquering the wilderness, they were living in great physical discomfort, suffering constant illness, and dying young, especially the women, who were worn out by incessant childbirth and endless chores.

The full impact of the continuing political, social, and economic changes was felt in the 1830s. The constant movement of people and the population increase deepened the strains. Universal suffrage, the mass party, and the political machine required a different adjustment to government. Small factories were expanding in all directions, disrupting direct personal dealings among craftsmen, mechanics, and customers. Thousands of volunteer workers were circulating antislavery petitions, and for the first time substantial numbers of women "found a satisfying mode of civic activity in which they could engage with reasonable propriety" (Elkins 1959:187).

It was a sharply upturning prosperity situation with a thousand new alternatives for action; it was at the same time one in which limits were being broken everywhere, in which traditional expectations were disrupted profoundly—a classic instance of that tension-producing state . . . named "anomie" (Elkins 1959:165).

As the physical frontier contracted near the end of the century, the frontiers of industry, technology, and science expanded in the cities. But the migrations to the city began before the supply of land was exhausted.

When cars, movies and radios become essentials of the accepted standard of living, subsistence farming is repugnant even to the starving. Measured, therefore, against this concept of a changing . . . standard of living . . . the lure of the land began in Tudor England before there was any available, and ceased in the United States before the supply gave out (Potter 1958:159).

The great technological inventiveness of Americans and their speedy adjustment to the machine age have been attributed to the resourcefulness and adaptability which developed out of the frontier experience, as well as to the absence of a traditional stratified society.

The frontier liberated the American spirit. It developed generosity and radiant vitality, together with a restlessness which was both good and ill, but did certainly bring with it a resiliency of mind, fluidity of idea and of society, a willingness for bold experiment (C. Kluckhohn 1965:210).

Dominant Child-Rearing Values and Practices

The value system which derived from Puritanism and the frontier was reflected in the theories and methods of child rearing. The goal was to produce adults who would function effectively in a competitive, aggressive, striving, and achieving society. But simultaneous training for independence, self-reliance, and individualism, on the one hand, and obedience, submission, and sensual repression, on the other, created major discontinuities. The strains resulting from these contradictions were mitigated, however, by the countertheme of indulgence and permissiveness that appeared in the early years of settlement. This countertheme became dominant in the 1940s when socioeconomic changes and new knowledge in the social sciences shifted the emphases for adult functioning.

Calvinist child rearing was based on the tenets of infant conversion and the "natural depravity" of the child. Infant conversion demonstrated that a child who accepted religious truth was becoming an independent moral being, on the road to salvation. The "inherently depraved" child could be saved from sin only by complete obedience to strict parental guidance, achieved by breaking the child's will.

The frontier experience, however, weakened the traditional European patriarchal family and the father's role as instructor, disciplinarian, and religious head of the family. A new type of democratic family relationship emerged in which the son addressed his father with "mingled freedom, familiarity, and affection" (Tocqueville 1956:231). By the end of the eighteenth century the American family and school already appeared to the English traveler to be child oriented and overly permissive.

They [children] were rarely punished at home, and strict discipline was not tolerated in the schools. . . . as he [the child] could not be punished in the school, he learned to regard his teacher as an inferior and to disregard all law and order (Lipset 1967:93).

In the 1820s a substantial body of American literature on child rearing began to appear. This new concern reflected confidence in the ability to mold the child so that he would realize parental ambitions. It also reflected the growing belief in the perfectibility of man under proper guidance, and in his capacity to master the universe and control the future. Perhaps even more significant, as traditional patterns broke down, parents sought direction on how to rear their children. This reliance on expert opinion for child-rearing practices was thenceforth to characterize American parents in a society that changed continually.

The child-rearing literature represented the dominant middle-class values, deriving from Calvinist theory, which asserted that the carefully reared child would become "a moral, honest, religious, independent individual who would take his proper place in society" (Sunley 1955: 151). The Calvinists claimed that the child's character was formed during his first six years, principally by the mother, who was thus held responsible for the child's future life, his fate after death, the welfare of the nation, and indeed for the whole human race. The widespread opposition to the women's rights movement that was beginning to develop was based on the asserted primacy of woman's role as mother and wife, which demanded wholehearted and exclusive dedication to the family.

The literature stressed the Calvinist belief that the child's will had to be broken, and that this could be achieved by a policy of nonindulgence and strict training. In practice, however, foreign observers pointed out that in the American family children were the center of attention. According to Trollope, "they eat and drink as they please; they are never punished; they are never banished, snubbed and kept in the background, as children are with us" (Lipset 1967:92).

The literature recommended educational activities to arouse the curiosity and encourage the independence of the preschool child. Harriet Martineau said that the American child did indeed have "the best possible early discipline; that of activity and self-dependence" (Lipset 1967:92). But "parents apparently often forced infants and young children to perform beyond their physical or mental level" (Sunley 1955: 156). And British travelers observed that the precocity, maturity and independence of American children were achieved "at the loss of parental control" (Lipset 1967:92).

The literature generally emphasized early toilet training to establish "habits of cleanliness and delicacy," for lack of sphincter control was viewed with disgust and disapproval. "Some mothers expressed the feeling that success in early toilet training was to the credit of the child and themselves" (Sunley 1955:157), and personal cleanliness, neatness, and orderliness were equated with morality.

The early literature expressed the Calvinist horror of autoeroticism. Parents accepted the views of European doctors that masturbation led to "disease, insanity, and even death," and the upper classes blamed the habit on "servants, slaves or depraved children" (Sunley 1955: 157, 158). Parents and nurses were urged to watch closely over children's play and were warned against sexually suggestive behavior.

Incorporated into Northern reformism in the 1830s and 1840s was a new child-rearing philosophy which opposed Calvinist views. This philosophy enjoined parents to be gentle, consistent, and firm with children, and urged parents to help the child fulfill his needs and potentialities by the use of encouragement and reward. Corporal punishment, isolation, and shaming were to be shunned because they did not create the desired results. Horace Mann and Henry Barnard campaigned for local school boards, professional teacher training, and free secular public schools, which they believed would put an "end to the philosophy of *Authority, Force, Fear and Pain that indissolubly associated together the ideas of Childhood and Punishment*" (Handlin 1963:252).

An Englishman who visited schools in New York state in 1833, however, found no signs of "authority, force, fear and pain."

The pupils are entirely independent of their teachers. No correction, no coercion, no manner of restraint is permitted to be used. . . . Corporal punishment has almost disappeared from American day schools; and would meet with reprehension from the parents and perhaps retaliation from his scholars (Lipset 1967:32).

By 1860 the new educational program was well under way, and teachers were being trained in normal schools. Women teachers were replacing men in elementary schools, mothers were replacing fathers as disciplinarians in the home, and the use of corporal punishment was everywhere diminishing.

But an analysis of *Infant Care,* the Children's Bureau bulletin, from 1914 to 1951, showed the strength and persistence of Puritanism in American child rearing, as well as increasingly dominant middle-class theme of permissiveness in the latter part of the period.

Shifts in the pattern of infant care—especially on the part of middle-class mothers—show a striking correspondence to the changes in practices advocated in successive editions of U. S. Children's Bureau bulletins and similar sources of expert opinion (Bronfenbrenner 1958:425).

The 1914 edition of *Infant Care* urged mothers to battle ceaselessly against the "child's sinful nature," especially his "strong and dangerous impulses" toward thumb-sucking and masturbation. The child's needs were sharply distinguished from his desires, and if his needs were satisfied his cries should go unheeded or he would become a tyrant. Playing with the baby was unwholesome and bad for his nerves.

In the editions of 1929 and 1938, play had become less dangerous, but it was to be limited to certain times of the day. Reflecting the emphasis on efficiency and time-orientation in the business world, the child was to be raised "by the clock." He should be weaned and toilet-trained early, with great firmness and regularity, for child rearing was regarded as a contest for domination between parents and children. When the child masturbated, however, he was no longer to be restrained, but diverted.

The 1942 edition was drastically revised, permissiveness becoming the principal theme. Later weaning and toilet training were now recommended, the baby's erotic and dominating impulses having weakened considerably. Thumb-sucking was to be accepted, but when the child masturbated he was still to be diverted so that he would not use his body as a plaything. The baby's needs and desires were now equated, and the dichotomy between the good and the pleasurable was bridged. Indulgence would no longer make a tyrant of the child. Play was now wholesome physical and exploratory activity, and mothers were urged to incorporate play and singing into their routines so that they would be "fun" for parent and child alike. The father re-entered the child-rearing scene, for children were to be enjoyed by both parents. In fact, "parents are promised that having children will keep them together, keep them young, and give them fun and happiness. . . . It seems difficult here for anything to become permissible without becoming compulsory. Play, having ceased to be wicked . . . now becomes a new duty" (Wolfenstein 1955:173).

The child-rearing values of the 1940s reflected the trend in adult amusement, which was being "increasingly divested of puritanical associations of wickedness" (Wolfenstein 1955:174). Now there was concern about whether the impulse toward fun was sufficiently strong.

While gratifications of forbidden impulses traditionally aroused guilt, failure to have fun currently occasions lowered self-esteem. One is likely to feel inadequate, impotent, and also unwanted (Wolfenstein 1955:174).

"Fun morality" was also prominent in the 1951 edition of *Infant Care,* but boredom crept in as a new reason for infant autoeroticism. And restraints on the child's exploratory activities and tendency to dominate were again advocated to keep him out of trouble. The 1957 edition of Spock's *Baby and Child Care* also discussed the conflict between "love" and "limits."

If the parent can determine in which respects she may be too permissive and can firm up her discipline, she may . . . be delighted to find that her child becomes not only better behaved but much happier. Then she can really love him better, and he in turn responds (p. 326).

By this time the middle-class parent was typically using "love-oriented" discipline, which relied for its effect on the child's fear of loss of love. The psychologists were insisting that frequent physical punishment tended to increase, not decrease aggressive behavior. Middle-class parents were therefore using physical punishment far less and relying more on reason, appeals to guilt, expressions of disappointment, and isolation. They also trained the child in a more leisurely fashion, having extended their time perspective.

But despite the greater lenience about "oral behavior, toilet accidents, sex and aggressiveness," middle-class parents had "not relaxed their high levels of expectations for ultimate performance." Moreover, their disciplinary methods were "likely to be effective in evoking the behavior desired in the child" (Bronfenbrenner 1958:414, 415).

the compelling power of these practices . . . is probably enhanced by the more permissive treatment accorded to middle-class children in the early years of life. . . . The more love present in the first instance, the greater the threat implied in its withdrawal (Bronfenbrenner 1958:419).

The changing role requirements for adults had been leading to different emphases in child rearing. In a society of small firms and small-scale government, individual achievement grows out of strict upbringing. But when large corporations and massive government bureaucracies predominate, permissive training is required to produce adults who adjust easily and are skilled in interpersonal communication (Miller and Swanson 1958). A likeable personality, once irrelevant to achievement, had become an important asset in the business world (Riesman 1950). Entertainment became a part of business relations, and the demarcation between work and play was blurred.

Moreover, as the economy changed from production to consumption, the theme of hedonistic gratification replaced asceticism in order to increase consumer activity. The concept of boredom, introduced into the 1951 *Infant Care,* no doubt reflected the thirst for novelty and the rapid obsolescence of consumer goods, stimulated by the communications media, particularly television.

Margaret Mead's early analysis of American child-rearing values and practices seems still to be valid. According to Mead (1942), the American child learns very soon that his place in the world depends on his family's status, as determined by the father's occupation and income, the kind of house he owns and the car he drives. The child learns that only personal achievement, comparatively evaluated, makes him worthy of love, and he is filled with anxiety about his ability to achieve enough to earn and retain parental love. "So the young American starts life with a tremendous impetus towards success" (p. 91). Since sibling rivalry is expressed by competition for parental approval of personal achievement, a boy finds it less stressful to choose a career which is different from that of his father and siblings. Because it is difficult to compare achievement in dissimilar fields, income becomes the measure of success. Only the child who is intelligent, beautiful, and strong has the assurance which derives from unconditional approval and can, in turn, transmit this assurance to his own children.

Absolute values for judging children have disappeared in the United States because the content and methods of learning change very rapidly to accord with the speed of technological change. Thus, American parents reject the guidance of their own mothers and fathers, and sharply enforce conformity to the norms of the community in which they happen to be living. They evaluate their children's performance by comparing it with that of the neighbors' children. What counts is the child's place on the normal distribution curve. When pediatricians, psychologists, and schools offer only a relative standard, parents punish and reward in its name. The American child is encouraged to be "brighter, stronger, more aggressive, more successful" than his parents, and he learns to boast as "a necessary precautionary measure, as he tries to live up to an unknown demand upon his unknown strength" (Mead 1942:155).

American values about aggression are ambivalent. Boys are taught to repress aggression but at the same time they are trained to defend themselves when someone else starts the fight. Americans emphasize the rules of fair play less than the English because they must learn to evaluate quickly each new situation as it comes up. They know far less what to expect because of the

confused, turbulent, unpatterned quality of American life, . . . part of it . . . due to the mixture of different standards of handling aggression, part of it symbolic, so that all those groups against which one is discriminating, Negroes, Puerto Ricans, Foreigners, Orientals, become invested with that hostility which we have shown them, and seem dangerous and threatening (Mead 1942:149).

In the United States, the small nuclear family, with its few strong ties to extended kin, is vitally important to each member, and a parent's death may have a catastrophic effect on a child. "The fact that two parents are all the anchors he has in a world which is otherwise vague and shifting, overemphasizes the tie and brings it into question" (Mead 1942:85).

American parents behave as if they have all the virtues their children must acquire, endowing them with a conscience and a sense of guilt. But when the adolescent finds his parents wanting, he "faces the greatest spiritual dilemma of growing up in this culture." He then begins the quest for the parental substitute, for that which is better than himself. For even when the parents prove to be fallible, "the belief that there is something better, wiser, stronger, freer, truer, survives their downfall" (Mead 1942:133, 134). And the belief in progress is reborn in each generation.

Inequality: The Great Contradiction

De Toqueville noted that while Americans pressed strongly for freedom, "for equality their passion is ardent, insatiable, incessant, invincible" (1956:192). Yet from the beginning of settlement this primary American value was violated, and the condition of inequality was forcibly thrust upon large groups of people. In each situation of inequality—the theft of lands from the Indians and their subjugation, the enslavement of the Africans, discrimination against the immigrant minorities—the economic motive was stronger than the ideal. But in each case the ideal was sufficiently vital and persistent that the naked economic motive had to be rationalized.

THE INDIANS

The sovereign rights of the Indians were affirmed by the English courts at the beginning of colonization, and from time to time thereafter by the Americans. At first the natives and the immigrants were friendly. The Indians came to the rescue of the starving colonists and shared with them their techniques for surviving in the wilderness.

The English hoped that the Indians would reveal stores of gold such as had been found in Mexico and Peru. They desperately needed labor and they tried to convert the natives to Christianity. But the Indians had no gold, and at the first attempts to force them to work they fled into the forest. They rejected Christianity, for conversion meant the abandonment not only of their gods but of their whole way of life. Soon they began to resent the intrusion upon their lands. "In time their resentment mounted at the pushy, crowding strangers who seemed never satisfied with what they had and were incomprehensible in their limitless claims for land." Tension increased until it broke out into open hostility and savage warfare on both sides. The settlers became embittered by the loss of life they suffered, and "by the damages wilderness fighting compelled them to inflict" (Handlin 1963:64, 65).

The English yeomen and artisans had lived in cleared open spaces for centuries and their folklore showed their dread of the English forests. Amid the hardships and terrors of the New World their latent fears erupted, and they looked upon the Indians as the embodiment of "the dreadful dehumanizing power of the wilderness." (Handlin 1963: 65). Outraged by their "indecent habits and heathenish practices, . . . their wild and dissolute behavior," the puritanical English and their American descendants felt they were justified when they took away the Indian lands by any means they could. President Thomas Jefferson himself suggested one method of land-grabbing to the governor of the Indiana Territory:

It was the duty of the Indians to "withdraw themselves to the culture of a small piece of land." Soon they would "perceive how useless to them were extensive forests" and would be willing "to pare them off from time to time in exchange for the necessities for their farms and families." That inclination could be promoted by setting up trading houses where "the good and influential among them would run up debts beyond what they could pay" and then would be willing "to lop them off" by a cession of lands (Handlin 1963:158).

Many Americans experienced acute mental discomfort about tactics which might be expected of European despots, but were not appropriate to the free people of a republic. But they found rationalizations.

Wistfully, Americans told themselves that the Indians really did not like it where they were. . . . It was in their own self-interest that they should go, until some future time when they would be able to associate, as they should, on equal terms with other Americans (Handlin 1963:159).

Except for the Quakers, some missionaries, and the fur-trappers and pioneers who fraternized and intermarried with them, the immigrants treated the Indians and their cultures with contempt and hostility. And it had soon become clear that the white man's culture brought them only disease and vice. In 1803, Congress appropriated $3,000 "to civilize and educate the heathens." After 1815, when cotton reigned supreme, "the callous removal of the five civilized Indian nations from Georgia opened the way into . . . Alabama and Mississippi" (Handlin 1963:211). In 1819, Congress appropriated an annual fund of $10,000 to civilize the Indians.

One of the most tragic features of our own dealings with the American Indians has been the constant changes in policy which, together with tribal removals, have rendered the adaptations which they successively developed successively unworkable (Linton 1940:519).

The Indians fought desperately for their lands and their cultures for 300 years, the entire period being marked by "broken promises, bloody wars and deceptive treaties" (Handlin 1963:159). In the end the conquered Indians were placed on government reservations. Until 1933 the government continued its policy of forcible assimilation by fractionalizing Indian lands, by attempting to "civilize" and Christianize the Indians, and by the compulsory education of Indian children in government boarding schools. Only about 35 years ago did a new policy emerge to permit the Indians to manage their own affairs, govern themselves, develop their tribal resources, and practice their native religions. But government paternalism, impatient with what it regards as the slow pace of Indian progress, continues to intervene in Indian life.

The temptation to be directive and to do things for Indians rather than patiently to encourage them to achieve autonomy has frequently suppressed Indian initiative and strengthened the bonds of dependency (Mason 1955:1273).

The bitter legacy from the past is revealed in the present status of the American Indian.

His average annual income is one-half the amount which has been determined to be the general poverty level for the poor in the United States. He can expect to live to age 42. His segregation from the rest of society makes the Negro's degree of acceptance look good. The level of unemployment among his people is seven or eight times that of his nation's average unemployment. He suffers more from poor health, malnutrition and ignorance than does any other ethnic group in the country (Will and Vatter eds. 1965:163).

SLAVERY

During the first half-century of settlement in North America, the planters in Virginia and Maryland preferred white indentured servants to black slaves, and "occasional laws in the colonies attempted to prohibit or discourage the importation of Africans" (Handlin 1963:78). But when the Royal Africa Company lost its monopoly on slave trading near the end of the seventeenth century, independent slave traders, eager to broaden the market, offered liberal credit to buyers and made slaves readily available. The modern form of the plantation spread to those regions raising products which profited from large-scale investment in land, labor, and machinery, and after 1700, profits were plowed back into the plantations so that they could be expanded.

Not only did the slaves produce crops, but they were bred and also reproduced themselves. The planters in Virginia and Maryland, who found no advantage in using slave labor to grow tobacco, made good profits by raising and selling slaves to the colonies that grew rice, indigo, and cotton. So that black people could be transformed into production units for purchase or sale, slave codes defined blacks and their descendants as chattels and deprived them of all human rights and legal redress.

By contrast, the slave laws in the Latin American colonies assumed the humanity of slaves, according to Elkins, and granted them rights to marry freely, to seek another master when they were brutalized, to own property, to participate equally in the dominant religion, and to buy their freedom. All these rights were absent in North America, where slavery developed in a way that made it "unique among all such systems known to civilization" because no institutions existed, said Elkins, that were powerful enough to check and regulate it. The dynamism of capitalism was breaking the transplanted European traditions, permitting only those institutions to develop which helped, or did not impede, the individual in his drive for economic achievement. "With the full development of the plantation there was nothing . . . to prevent unmitigated capitalism from becoming unmitigated slavery" (Elkins 1959:42, 49).

According to Harris, however, the American Constitution expressed "a general Northern and enlightened Southern belief that slavery was an institution that was incompatible with the laws and traditions of civilized Englishmen." At the end of the eighteenth century, many Southerners viewed slavery as "uneconomic, morally dubious, and a burden on both the slaveholder and the community," and Washington, Randolph, and others made sporadic attempts at emancipation. But after the War of 1812 the demand for cotton and slaves increased so sharply that any Southern hostility to slavery disappeared, and Southerners found reasons to justify it. The Latin American slaveowners, Church, and state also actively opposed literacy and individual initiative

among the slaves in order to ensure a docile labor force. "The slav-
ocracy in both the Latin and the Anglo-Saxon colonies held the whip
hand not only over the slaves but over the agents of civil and eccle-
siastical authority" (Harris 1964:81).

Harris accounted for the different treatment of the slaves in Latin
and North America in terms of the different settlement experiences in
each area. With a manpower shortage in the Iberian Peninsula, comparatively few men left to colonize the New World. There was, in fact,
little incentive to settlement, since, throughout Latin America the sugar
planters had monopolized the best land in the lowlands, and a settled
native Indian population lived in the highlands. Faced with a chronic
labor shortage, the slaveowners were forced to create a class of free
half-castes to perform economic and military functions for which slave
labor could not be used.

On the other hand, the prospect of buying land at very low prices
after working off the passage debt brought the excess labor of England
to North America, and for almost the first century the population of
the English colonies was overwhelmingly white.

Because the influx of Africans and the appearance of mulattoes in the
United States occurred only *after* a large intermediate class of whites had
already been established, there was in effect no place for the freed slave,
. . . mulatto or Negro, to go (Harris 1964:89).

After the Civil War, the white middle and lower classes emphasized
discrimination by race in order to monopolize the better positions for
themselves in a rapidly expanding economy. But when slavery was
abolished in Latin America, the mulattoes and blacks vastly outnumbered the poor whites, and the peaceful relationships between the races
were due primarily to economic stagnation, with "very little of a significant nature to struggle over" (Harris 1964:96). Thus race was de-
emphasized in favor of class discrimination.

Immediately after the Civil War, the embittered Southerners bent all
their energies to restoring the old order. Those who had once held
power quickly regained it, substituted peonage for slavery and, backed
by the Ku Klux Klan and the Black Codes, established the political,
economic, and social inferiority of the blacks. The black people had no
choice but to submit, for the North resumed its own affairs, satisfied
that it had saved national unity and freed the slaves. The outcome of
the war cast doubts on the idea of human perfectibility and on the
ability of the government to bring about social justice.

NATIVISM AND ANGLO-CONFORMITY

"Anglo-conformity," the predominant attitude of Americans toward immigrants since earliest colonial times, demands "the complete renunciation of the immigrant's ancestral culture in favor of the behavior and values of the Anglo-Saxon core group" (Gordon 1964:85). The early colonists had contempt for the Indian host cultures, suppressed those of the Africans, and regarded the French and Spanish as representatives of the "Romish Whore of Babylon" (Handlin 1963:65). Although the peoples of northern and western Europe were not very different from the British, even Benjamin Franklin was suspicious of those who, like the Pennsylvania Germans, preserved their own customs and language. Both Washington and Jefferson expressed doubts about "the effects of mass immigration on American institutions" (Gordon 1964:90). In 1818 John Quincy Adams unequivocally expressed the slogan that still erupts from many Americans when their institutions are criticized:

if they [immigrants] cannot accommodate themselves to the character, moral, political and physical, of this country with all its compensating balances of good and evil, the Atlantic is always open to them to return to the land of their nativity (Gordon 1964:94).

The arrival of large numbers of poverty-stricken Irish Catholics after the potato famines in the 1840s aroused anxiety about the spread of "popery," and culminated during the 1850s in the anti-Catholic campaigns of the Know-Nothing Party. Commenting on the activities of this party, Abraham Lincoln wrote:

As a nation, we began by declaring that *"all men are created equal."* We now practically read it, "all men are created equal, except negroes." When the Know-Nothings get control, it will read "all men are created equal, except negroes, *and foreigners and Catholics."* When it comes to this, I should prefer emigrating to some country where they make no pretense of loving liberty (Gordon 1964:93).

After the Civil War the tremendous industrial expansion and continued settlement of the West required additional population, and the millions of immigrants who poured into the country were in general favorably received. The immigrants settled into the ghettos where their relatives were already established, formed associations to help one another, and "preserved the folk wisdom that had proved efficacious in the past" (Handlin 1963:283).

The cities grew not only from the influx of immigrants, but also from the very many young people who were leaving the farms. The native migrants pinched and scraped so that they could buy a house in the suburbs to be with their own kind, and "the birth rate among these Americans fell by about thirty percent between 1860 and 1900." But "social mobility destroyed the stability of the ghettos whether in the slums or in the suburbs" (Handlin 1963:284, 285).

Postwar scientific discoveries shook American fundamentalism, and the theories about the evolution of species were socially disruptive. The concept of separate and unequal races was used to justify slavery and segregation and to account for the failure of Reconstruction. Acting on the racist doctrines, the courts nullified the guarantees of the Four-teenth Amendment.

Good Christians no longer had to consider mankind a unity; after 1860 they could think in terms of distinct races, each with its own inherent biological traits, separate and unequal. The new understanding helped account for anomalies in the American social situation; . . . and it offered many people an escape from emotional tension (Handlin 1963:283).

Discrimination against anyone of different color—the Indians, the Chinese—was now legitimized. The Haymarket riots created fear of foreign radicals. Municipal reformers began to blame the immigrants for the crime, poverty, and political corruption in the cities, and Ameri-cans now found "racial differences" among whites. New Englanders formed the Immigration Restrictive League. Some Populist Party mem-bers inveighed against the economic power of the Jews. The American Protective Association attacked Irish Catholics. Labor leaders discrim-inated against Italians and Slavs.

Beset by the drastic changes resulting from increased industrializa-tion and urbanization, Americans searched desperately for stability and identity. They tried to find one another by excluding the alien, and the concept of "Americanism" emerged, to be integrated into the national consciousness by ritual and ceremonial. The children of the immigrants also rejected the foreign origins of their parents as a stigma that held them back.

Between 1900 and 1917, 12 million immigrants arrived, mainly from southern and eastern Europe. After 1900 the Jews faced a virulent anti-Semitism which barred or limited their access to various types of employment, residential areas, the universities, and the professions. Discrimination increased against all Catholics, not only the Irish. Amer-icans in the midwest and on the Pacific Coast also joined the Ku Klux Klan, and its membership rose to 4 million. Prohibition became the

rallying symbol of those striving to preserve the "purity" of the republic. "At no time in American history were southern race dogmas so
widely accepted throughout the entire nation as in the early years of
the twentieth century" (Elkins 1959:13). By depriving so many people
of equal opportunity, discrimination served the dual purpose of lessen-
ing economic competition and defining the group. It protected "Americans" against "outsiders," and gave the "Americans" pride in their
own "superiority."

"Americanism" flourished at a time when political and economic
"progressivists" were attacking the trusts and the power and privileges
of great wealth. Magazines of the period carried both muckraking articles
and articles declaring the superiority of Nordics and the inferiority of
most other peoples. The writings of a contemporary educator exemplify
the movement to strip the immigrants of their ethnic cultures:

Our task is to break up these groups . . . to assimilate these people as a
part of our American race, and to implant in their children, so far as can
be done, the Anglo-Saxon conception of righteousness, . . . and to awaken
in them a reverence for our democratic institutions (Gordon 1964:98).

By 1900 the university had become the medium for certifying culture
and science, and from the new intellectual stronghold flowed disparate
currents which influenced American thought. On the one hand, his-
torians and amateur scientists loudly proclaimed that the greater fertility of the southern and eastern European immigrants was smothering
the Nordics. On the other hand, scholars like Franz Boas, W. I.
Thomas, and William Graham Sumner disseminated the view that culture and society, not race or nationality, determined the condition of
men. As far back as the 1890s, settlement house workers were pleading
for cultural pluralism and for recognition of the actual and potential
contribution of the ethnic cultures to American life.

But the scientific opposition to the nativist doctrines and practices
was not to gain popular acceptance for another generation. World
War I increased the pressures on immigrants to "Americanize." Wood-
row Wilson stated in 1915 that "a man who thinks of himself as belonging to a particular national group in America has not yet become an
American" (Gordon 1964:101). Concomitantly, the increasingly bureaucratic government began to encroach on civil liberties. During World
War I, the first victims were women suffragists who were arrested and
jailed for picketing.

The outcome of the war and the events that took place in postwar
Europe accelerated the suppression of nonconformity in the United

States. "Reds" were hunted down and many were deported or jailed. The Sacco-Vanzetti trial showed that the poor, dissenters, and the foreign-born could not get a fair trial.

Americans did not recognize the importance of the ethnic community in helping to acculturate the immigrants.

The self-contained communal life of the immigrant colonies served . . . as a kind of decompression chamber in which the newcomers could, at their own pace, make a reasonable adjustment to the new forces of a society vastly different from that which they had known in the Old World (Gordon 1964:106).

In the normal course of events the ethnic cultures could survive only marginally because immigrant children were exposed, with great intensity, to American models in the schools and the communications media. But although Americanization brought advantages in the job market, it did not open the door to friendship with members of the dominant culture. Frequently the result was delinquency when children were alienated from the family and the parental culture but were not permitted to integrate socially with the broader society.

Not until the depression of the 1930s was the tide of racism and nativism, which had prevailed for half a century, reversed by the hope provided by the New Deal and the unionization of mass-production workers. Now people became more attentive to the social scientists who were demonstrating the oneness of the human species. And as Americans fought together in World War II, "they recoiled as one from the revelations in the Nazi extermination camps of the logical corollary of the doctrine of Aryan supremacy" (Handlin 1963:396). However, the wholesale internment of the Japanese and Japanese-Americans during the war "revealed that in times of acute stress racist premises could again direct the hand of official action" (Gordon 1964:102).

After the war, young married people all over the country moved in unprecedented numbers to the suburbs, impelled by fear of the violence, crime and dirt of the city slums, which they blamed on the new minorities, the blacks and the Latin American peoples. But the young suburbanites began to cherish their own religious heritage, for "the descendants of the immigrants, now in their third generation, endowed the ethnic group with sanctity, wholeness and security" (Handlin 1963:408).

The colored minorities were entering the economic mainstream at a far slower pace than the European immigrants. Rural blacks moving to the cities in the South and the North were given only the lowest-paid jobs, and the language difference increased the difficulties of the Puerto

Ricans and the Mexican-Americans. While the economy grew in all directions during and after World War II, the colored minorities were excluded from most of the benefits. Technological development increased the number of white-collar and technical jobs, which required greater education and training. But it also decreased semiskilled and unskilled employment, and the untrained minorities became poorer as the rest of the nation grew richer.

The black man who had fought in World War II was determined to share at last in the American heritage of equal opportunity, civil rights, and individual dignity. Inspired also by the formation of the new African nations, black people began to take pride in their black identity and to participate actively in protest movements. Although education and employment opportunities improved and more blacks moved into the middle class, the gains were made too slowly, and soon the movement for equality was to embrace the theme of violence as well as nonviolence. With the example of the black power movement, other groups of second-class citizens—Mexican-Americans, Puerto Ricans, Indians, youth, women—entered the economic, political, and civil rights arena.

CHAPTER 9

Contemporary American Working-Class Values

Sociologists divide the American working class into two major group-ings, "old" and "new," in terms of socioeconomic status and life pat-terns. The vast majority of Puerto Rican migrants in New York City are members of the "new" working class, whose values and ways of life are "variations upon the theme of the stable working-class pattern" (S. M. Miller and Riessman 1964:27). Many of the values of the stable or "old" working class appear to contradict the dominant middle-class values.

The apparent contradictions in the American value system seem to be a natural consequence of a complex, heterogeneous, industrialized society, but they have led some scholars to characterize American culture as schizoid and inherently dualistic (Bain 1935:266–76; Laski 1948). According to Cora Du Bois (1955:1232–1233), however, such "oppositional propositions" are "spurious" and represent "recurrent dilemmas in logic and ethics" in western European culture, which are fostered by the structure of the Indo-European languages. "No viable value system . . . can entertain logical contraries," writes Du Bois. Values "strain for consistency" as social structures and institutions change.

. . . the viability of a value system does not rest exclusively on its internal coherence. It must also manifest a considerable degree of congruence with the situational context within which it exists. Changes in value systems will result, therefore, from the strain for consistency not only within the value system but also between values and situational factors (Du Bois 1955:1239).

A number of scholars have pointed out the dynamic relationships between values and social process. "Alternative value patterns," says

133

Goldschmidt, are institutionalized in social structures "to prevent organized resistance against the dominant values" (1960:431). Variant patterns are permitted in societies to mitigate the strains created by the dominant values. The variant patterns function to maintain the system "often over a very long time period, without serious disruptions," and they are, "therefore, the central feature of the structure of culture" (F. Kluckhohn and Strodtbeck 1961:43).

Opler conceived of "themes and counterthemes" as "the key to the equilibrium achieved in a culture." Counterthemes restrain the "extreme and unimpeded expression" of themes and are "the limiting factors, the circumstances . . . which control the number, force, and variety of a theme's expressions" (1945:201).

The complex interrelationships between the dominant and variant values of both old and new working classes in the United States arise out of their respective adaptations to changing economic, political, and social structures.

The Value of Work

The reciprocal influence between attitudes toward work and specific religious affiliation is notable in the United States, which is still a highly religious country. A 1968 Gallup Poll showed that 98 percent of Americans believe in God; 73 percent, in a life after death; 65 percent, in hell; 60 percent, in the devil. The corresponding percentages for Britain were 77, 38, 23 and 21. The American precentages exceed "the percentages with such beliefs in 11 other nations."[1]

Most members of the middle and upper classes have always been Protestant, but white blue-collar workers tend to be Catholic far more than Protestant, although an increasing number of Catholics is moving upward. The relatively recent immigration of Catholics and their entrance into the economic order at a fairly low level does not appear to account for their preponderance in the working class. Comparisons of white Protestants and Catholics who began life in the middle class and as sons of farmers, show that "Catholics more often than Protestants three out of four times" wound up as blue-collar workers, and that "the Protestants rose to or stayed in the ranks of the upper middle class more often" (Vernon 1964:319). The processes of Americanization and urbanization appear to increase the differences between Protestants and Catholics.

---

[1] *The New York Times,* December 25, 1968.

According to their proportion in the several classes, either white Protestants or Jews are ranked first or second, Catholics are third, and black Protestants, fourth. The higher socioeconomic status of Jews and white Protestants is attributed to the fact that they have very consistently

identified themselves with the individualistic competitive patterns of thought and action linked with the middle class, and historically associated with the Protestant Ethic or its secular counterpart, the spirit of capitalism. By contrast, Catholics and Negro Protestants have more often been associated with the collectivistic, security-oriented working-class patterns of thought and action historically opposed to the Protestant Ethic (Lenski 1961:100).

Meier and Bell, however, ascribe the lesser achievement of Catholics to their lack of opportunity rather than to their religious values. "In American society, opportunity is narrowed by race and nationality, physical handicaps, and sex, among other conditions" (1959:201).

Nevertheless, a reciprocal relationship does seem to exist between upward mobility and involvement in the white Protestant churches, but not in the Catholic Church. The Protestant sects in the United States, as in Puerto Rico, appeal primarily to blue-collar workers. Although the sects emphasize otherworldly rewards, they also encourage industriousness, frugality, deferred gratification, excellence in work performance—in short, the Puritan virtues necessary for worldly success. But when the blue-collar worker adopts these values and becomes upwardly mobile, he may leave the sects and affiliate with more traditional denominations.

In the Protestant ethic, self-respect and self-actualization are contingent on work, which is viewed as an end in itself. Hard work and striving are the keys to successful achievement, as measured by the degree of upward mobility attained by the individual. Under frontier conditions these assumptions were even more valid in the United States than in Europe, "labor was scarce, the returns from an individual's work were unusually high, and the opportunities to rise from a lower to a higher economic and social status were relatively constant" (Wright 1957:23).

The American nation was developed by mobility, both horizontal and vertical, and mobility continually undermined class lines. As obstacles to upward mobility increased, however, class lines hardened and variant values evolved. These, for most working-class people, are security, stability, compensatory consumption, and the search for excitement.

Even in periods of prosperity, skilled and semiskilled workers fear the "occasional layoffs of some duration, . . . episodes of recession, plant relocation, industry decline, strikes" (S. M. Miller and Riessman 1964:30) and the replacement of men by automated machines. The desire to rise to foreman, the only upgrading available to most blue-collar workers, is sharply limited by the loss of union protection in this position. The basic goal of the vast majority of blue-collar workers is "getting by" rather than "getting ahead."

In order to maintain family and social stability, the blue-collar worker now strongly resists long-distance geographical movement, except in depression periods. Moreover, such movement rarely offers him the vertical mobility that is the incentive of the white-collar man who moves. No more than 2 or 3 percent of blue-collar workers uproot themselves when a plant relocates, even when they know their economic situation will worsen if they "stay put."

The traditional American emphasis on business ownership as a means of achieving upward mobility and independence is expressed in the following formula:

any ambitious American youth with industry, average intelligence, and thrift can save enough money to start a small business and, if he has real initiative and ability, can develop it into a profitable business of considerable size (Mayer and Goldstein 1964:537).

However, nationwide polls and studies of the labor market and new small businesses, conducted between 1940 and 1960, showed that the typical white-collar worker now achieves upward mobility in a government bureaucracy or corporation, and "the desire to become a businessman has largely become a working-class dream" (Mayer and Goldstein 1964:549). Although blue-collar workers do go into business to achieve independence, they are motivated primarily by actual or imminent unemployment. Few anticipate substantial profits; most are satisfied with the same modest returns as they obtain from a job.

A longitudinal study of new small businesses, conducted from 1958 to 1960, showed that most blue-collar men went into the kind of business in which they were previously employed and that almost two-thirds failed within two years, a higher failure rate than for white-collar men. The blue-collar men failed because of inexperience in business management, lack of rational planning due to insufficient education, and capital investment that was too limited to sustain the business over emergency periods.

The high proportion of those who return to manual work, coupled with the fact that even those who stay in business are operating at economic levels which differ little from paid employment, raises grave doubts as to whether business ownership constitutes a channel of permanent upward mobility for more than a very small proportion of manual workers (Mayer and Goldstein 1964:549).

The fact that many workers in the last two decades have been able, because of installment buying, to obtain suburban homes, cars, and expensive appliances, is presented as proof of their middle-class values.[2] On the other hand, working-class consumer activity is regarded as compensation for blocked upward mobility (Chinoy 1952:453), or as an outlet for boredom in a humdrum life. And when blue-collar workers buy homes, it is not for middle-class status reasons, but to escape the domination of a landlord and to have a paid-up house for the non-earning retirement years (Handel and Rainwater 1964:39).

In an industrial society the work situation itself, according to Karl Marx, alienates the worker not only from the process and products of his work, but also from himself and others (1964:254). Contemporary social scientists have found this to be the case for large numbers of the middle class as well. The diminishing emphasis on individualism and the growing tendency of the suburban middle class to stress security more than hard work are "reactions to the strains associated with circumscribed opportunities and intense competition in the occupational sphere" (Mizruchi 1964:261). Furthermore, "standardization and automation are making robots of the middle-class worker," as well as the blue-collar worker:

in the white-collar spheres, as in industry, personal gratification as a result of work as an end in itself and also as a result of the products of one's efforts is a feeling enjoyed by the few rather than the many (Mizruchi 1964:259).

But it is factory work, above all, that is characterized as "inherently alienative." Automobile workers, for example, regard their work with "hatred, shame and resignation." The more they are exposed to middle-class values, the more degrading they find production-line work. But "it is not simply status-hunger that makes a man hate work that is mindless, endless, stupefying, sweaty, noisy, exhausting, insecure in its prospects, and practically without hope of advance" (Swados 1960:199). The devaluation of factory work is accompanied by "a false idealization of the white-collar job," particularly by blacks. At least for their children black workers want "prestige and power . . . in white-collar jobs and in the professions" (Purcell 1964:161). "Many Negro youngsters don't want the factory jobs even at $3.30 an hour to start. They want the white collar jobs that symbolize status in America."[3]

A comparative study of retired white-collar and blue-collar men

---

[2]Worker Loses His Class Identity, *Business Week,* July 11, 1959, p. 90.
[3]*The New York Times,* January 19, 1969, p. 5E.

showed that only a fourth of them regarded work positively, as a means of self-expression. Almost two-thirds, who valued work negatively, either missed nothing about their previous jobs or missed former associates. The white-collar man did not relate to society solely through his occupation, tended to have more self-esteem and to adjust better to retirement. Although the blue-collar workers placed a negative value or no value on work, their self-concept suffered when they retired. Even though they felt that they had accomplished nothing, "without their occupational roles as anchors, their lives fade into insignificance" (Loether 1964:529). The meaninglessness of work "is closely related to the meaninglessness of life to many American workers" (Purcell 1964:153).

The Protestant Ethic . . . seems a hopelessly irrelevant normative system in a culture of interlocked metropolises, international emporia, abstract world markets, and magisterial processes and ideas characterized by a vast secularism of value and expectation (Meadows 1964:459).

The meaning of work to the new working class derives from its marginal position in the economy, for it contains the largest proportion of unemployed and underemployed in an American society that is still work-oriented. The vast technological changes that are taking place are "further reducing employment opportunities for the displaced and for low-educated youth," and the income inequality between the poor and the rest of society "seems to be increasing" (S. M. Miller 1964a:3).

Automation in the rural south and in the agricultural sector of Puerto Rico is pushing the rural poor toward the large cities. But the metropolises, generating their own poor, are exerting no pull on the rural migrants, as they did during and after World War II. Now they do not need their labor and are not prepared to receive them. Thus the new working class, the urban poor, typically have "second-class economic and political citizenship," marked by

inadequate housing as they suffer the bulk of the ravages (and reap few of the benefits) of urban redevelopment, the poor schooling offered their children, the neglect of public services in their neighborhoods, the frequent callousness of the police and welfare departments, their bilking by merchants (S. M. Miller 1964a:8).

Although the child in the culture of poverty suffers from the chronic unemployment and underemployment in his family and community, the school orients him to the Protestant Ethic. The dichotomy between dominant values and the realities of life in the slums creates "work-value dissonant situations" that arouse tension and anxiety within the children. To reduce the dissonance, a new community, "in both the ecological and social-psychological sense, comes into existence in which new values are communicated and shared" (Schwartz and Henderson 1964:461). Work is devalued; techniques are invented to avoid working, and methods such as vice and crime are used to make money.

Such deviant behavior occurs in all social strata in the United States "when the individual has assimilated the cultural emphasis upon the goal without equally internalizing the institutional norms governing ways and means for its attainment." The fortunes made by the Robber Barons attest to the "strains toward institutionally dubious innovation" among the upper classes. A study of about 1,700 middle-class people in New York state revealed that "ninety-nine percent . . . confessed to having committed one or more of 49 offenses . . . each . . . being sufficiently serious to draw a maximum sentence of not less than a year." Many crimes committed by members of the middle and upper classes are not detected, and often go unpunished when they do come to light because the general American public expresses "reluctant admiration" for such "shrewd, smart and successful" people (Merton 1949:134–36).

It is true, however, that "the greatest pressures toward deviation are exerted upon the lower strata," given their lack of opportunity for advancement and "the American stigmatization of manual labor *which has been found to hold rather uniformly in all social classes*" (Merton 1949:136). A feudal system limits opportunity far more than the present American society, but deviant behavior takes place on a large scale

only when a system of cultural values extols, virtually above all else, certain *common* success-goals *for the population at large* while the social structure rigorously restricts or completely closes access to approved modes of reaching these goals *for a considerable part of the same population* (Merton 1949:137).

Unlawful acts, resistance to authority and risk-taking express variant values which originated in the early days of the frontier and are recurrent sanctified themes in the mass media, but they have become the dominant values of a certain proportion of the new working class. James Baldwin wrote that some of the black poor substitute crime for work as the only alternative. "Crime became real . . . not as *a* possibility but as *the* possibility. One would never defeat one's circumstances by working and saving one's pennies" (Baldwin 1962:59).

Some gains achieved through unemployment may become institutionalized in the culture of the "hard-core" poor, "a social grouping resistant to job opportunities, willing to accept an unemployment status as a way of life, and largely committed to values which deny the utility of employment" (Ferman 1964:514). Life is more predictable when people receive regular state aid than when they are irregularly employed. Landlords and shopkeepers can be paid out of a steady income, and creditors are less pressing.

Chronic unemployment and underemployment also bred the Black Power movement, which gives black youth an opportunity to release "frustrations and tensions stemming from unemployment experiences that is not open to unemployed white youth" (Ferman 1964:510).

As employment opportunities become available, some black and Spanish-speaking peoples must "unlearn" antiwork values. "The Puerto Ricans had not learned to strive, whereas Negroes had learned not to strive" (McCullens and Plant 1964:602). The attitudes of black people were learned in a work-value dissonant situation. The attitudes of Puerto Rican people were learned in a semifeudal Latin American society which discouraged the peasant from striving for upward mobility, and regarded work only as an instrument for survival, not an end in itself.

The Working-Class Family

The principal agency of acculturation for the Puerto Rican migrant in New York City is his immediate milieu, the working-class subculture. The American working class is divided not only into "old" and "new," but also into "upper" and "lower." The upper working class is itself often subdivided into two groups, traditional and modern, in terms of the differences in family and social life. The key to the understanding of the working class as a whole is the old, traditional, upper group, for the values of the other groups are "variations upon the theme of the stable working-class pattern" (S. M. Miller and Riessman 1964:27).

THE STABLE, TRADITIONAL, UPPER-LOWER FAMILY

Members of the old working class are likely to be white and Protestant, or second or third-generation Catholic, who work in comparatively highly paid, unionized, skilled and semiskilled occupations in the economic mainstream. Their lives center around the large extended family, which provides the principal goals of security and stability.

Economic and social relationships are frequently intertwined in the working-class extended family. Very often a youth chooses an occupation in which his father or another close relative is already working, thereby gaining entry into the same factory and the "closely controlled union" (Handel and Rainwater 1964:40). There appears to be "a greater continuity for the skilled than for most major occupational groupings" (Hamilton 1964:56). Members of the traditional working class make every effort to live close to parents, siblings, or other relatives, with whom they spend most of their social life. Mutual aid and cooperation within the extended family are the primary means for coping with instability.

But factors within the extended family also promote instability. These are "family discord, including divorce and desertion, intergenerational conflict, and the desire for excitement" (S. M. Miller and Riessman 1964:30). Class ranking and the divorce rate are inversely correlated in the United States and express "the generally greater marital instability in lower social strata" (Goode 1946:88). The causes are related to the frustrations arising from lesser work satisfaction and prestige, and from greater economic difficulties and insecurity, which are often displaced onto marital life. "This is especially likely in the United States, where the lack of rigid class definitions means that people cannot be easily content with their lot" (Goode 1946:88). Moreover, even the unionized worker is far more vulnerable than middle and upper-class people to automation, layoffs and unemployment. "His own pleasures are few enough, and his fears are great and growing. Threatened to the saturation point, he will often, in anger and impotence, strike back at his wife" (Sexton 1964:84).

Because of the forces that threaten him in the impersonal, competitive society, and his limited education and narrow social experiences, the traditional blue-collar worker generally believes in fate or luck. His "world view is one of pervasive anxiety, . . . sense of powerlessness and of insecurity," which he tries to decrease by a noncompetitive "network of highly personal relationships" with relatives and friends in similar circumstances. The reliance on personal relationships makes the working-class family extremely sensitive to the opinions of others in the same class and creates great pressures to conform to working-class mores. "Perhaps more than in any other class, the working class family looks horizontally for its norms and standards rather than outside or up to the next class" (Patterson 1964:78).

Stable working-class families want recognition only on a respectable "common man" level. The contents of a house are practical and utilitarian and are more important than the house itself. Except that "they seek to avoid slums or checkerboard neighborhoods, the socially significant address has little or no meaning for them" (Patterson 1964:78).

The family is patriarchal and sex roles are sharply segregated. In the United States as well as in Puerto Rico, the wife "sometimes knows nothing about her husband's work—what he does or even where his job is located." She may be hostile to his union because he spends so much time there. The husband often opposes the organization of women's auxiliaries as an invasion of his masculine stronghold, for "the union man all too frequently feels that a wife's place is at home." Most unions communicate with workers' wives mainly during strikes, when the women's support is a life-and-death issue. If wives are not informed about strike objectives and the money begins to run out, they may spark back-to-work movements. But when they do become involved in the union through the auxiliaries, they are often very enthusiastic and active, which "is threatening to men who have enough problems" (Sexton 1964:83–85).

Without union involvement the worker's wife is "a lonely, frightened, unhappy, frustrated cipher," who leads a life of "quiet desperation." Though deeply religious, she does not attend church regularly. Nor does she generally participate in the P.T.A. She is utterly dependent on her family, the neighborhood, and television. Most of all she relies on her husband, but tends to see him as "insensitive and inconsiderate," giving her "little affection or attention in payment for her drudgery," and generally treating her as an "object for his own personal gratification" (Sexton 1964:81–82).

The worker's wife must resort to installment buying for the necessary appliances and furniture, and she is guilt-stricken about the debts she incurs. "She is much more discontented with her financial status than is the middle-class woman" (Sexton 1964:83). A comparative study of working-class women in a lying-in clinic and patients of private obstetricians showed that the blue-collar women were more likely to view the future pessimistically and to have "a negative or inadequate self-image" (Rosengren 1964:337).

An analysis of sixteen studies of middle- and working-class child-rearing values and practices throughout the United States revealed that since the early 1940s working-class mothers have been less lenient than middle-class mothers in early child training. They were less likely to overlook offenses, more likely to use ridicule and withdrawal of privileges, and were less affectionate, egalitarian, and accepting of the child's desires and impulses. "The most consistent finding . . . is the more frequent use of physical punishment by working-class parents" (Bronfenbrenner 1958:419). However, a higher percentage of middle-class children were punished in some way, especially to prevent injury and danger. There was no class difference in the use of praise, except that working-class parents praised good behavior at the table more than the middle class.

The working-class family was not child-oriented, but parent-centered, and had taken over "the traditional middle-class virtues of cleanliness, conformity and control," with particular emphasis on ·obedience and respect for adults. The middle-class father had a warmer relationship with his children than the working-class father, and was "also likely to have more authority and status in family affairs." Although the working-class father demanded "compliance and control in his child," he was "himself more aggressive, expressive and impulsive than his middle-class counterpart" (Bronfenbrenner 1958:422–423).

Middle-class parents expected greater responsibility and a higher level of performance, especially in school. But while the working-class father shared middle-class aspirations, he had not yet learned how to achieve them either for himself or his children. "He has still to learn to wait, to explain, and to give and withhold his affection as the reward and price of performance" (Bronfenbrenner 1958:423).

A study of 100 American and 100 Swiss mothers, three-fourths in the upper-lower stratum, showed that the dominant values did influence American working-class mothers. The two groups of mothers were questioned about their values and practices in relation to stuttering, masturbation, lying, weaning, and bed-wetting, in the hope that attitudes toward these five "foci of disturbance," which were common in the United States and Switzerland, would reveal the interactions between the culture and the individual.

The American mothers at first gave the impression of being self-confident, aggressive, and vociferous, while the Swiss mothers appeared to be more placid and shy. During the interviews, however, "the American mother confirmed that she has set opinions less often and is much more inclined to depict herself as ignorant" (Jarecki 1961:341).

The Swiss mothers attached a strikingly greater significance to heredity and faulty upbringing as the causes of all the disturbances, and expressed great guilt about their child-rearing errors, while the American mothers appeared to deny parental responsibility for the problems. The Swiss mothers reared their children with the precision of a Swiss clock. They looked upon the child as a small adult who should adapt to his environment as quickly as possible. He was therefore expected to stop nursing, bedwetting, masturbating, and lying earlier than the American child, whose errors were more tolerated and who was permitted to remain young for a much longer time.

Both groups knew less about the reasons for masturbation than for the other disturbances, and agreed that the consequences could be sexual crimes, physical and mental damage, and so forth. "Thus a European tradition common to both peoples is [still] operative here" (Jarecki 1961:350). All the mothers regarded lying as morally wrong and as the most serious childhood problem, the majority stating that a child who lied would also steal, but the Swiss mothers saw lying as more reprehensible. They also condemned bed-wetting more severely than the Americans, and viewed it as rebellion against cleanliness and punctuality.

About two-thirds of the American mothers and half the Swiss mothers attributed stuttering to "psychic disturbance." "Almost 30% of both groups have had this or a similar speech problem" (Jarecki 1961:350), which was even more significant because several children were less than two years old and could not have stuttered. "The actual incidence of this symptom thus appears to be still greater." This incidence is so much greater than that found in surveys of stuttering in other European countries and the United States that it is very likely the mothers designated as speech problems many patterns which speech experts would regard as being within the normal range of speech.

The American mothers had read more about child rearing, "a consequence of the fact that popular presentations of child psychology are rather widely circulated in the United States, viz., Spock" (Jarecki 1961: 351), and this probably accounted, at least partially, for their greater permissiveness. By the late 1950s Spock had "joined the Bible on the working-class shelf" and, with increasing income and education, the working class was narrowing its "cultural lag" (Bronfenbrenner 1958:420).

According to S. M. Miller and Riessman, however, the traditional blue-collar worker "is not attracted to the middle-class style of life with its accompanying concern for status and prestige" (1964:29). In fact, "the best-off skilled workers are *least* like the middle class in attitudes and behavior" (Hamilton 1964:44) particularly in their minimal membership in organizations and their utilitarian approach to higher education. Although the traditional worker is concerned about his children's school work, "he feels estranged and alienated from the teacher and the school, as he similarly feels alienated from many institutions in our society" (S. M. Miller and Riessman 1964:29).

In the early 1960s about 40 percent of working-class youth dropped out of high school, and well over a third of the dropouts obtained only unskilled, irregular jobs. Perhaps 20 percent of working-class youth entered college, which "is a third of the over-all middle-class rate of college attendance." Also, "working-class youth are more likely than middle-class youth to leave college without the diploma" (S. M. Miller 1964c:123–126).

THE MODERN BLUE-COLLAR FAMILY

As their neighborhoods "are invaded by other ethnic groups or are torn down for redevelopment," working-class families may follow industry in its exodus to the suburbs. "The effect of these moves is to attenuate (both for the movers and for the stayers) the tight web of kin-based sociability that has traditionally characterized working-class life" (Rainwater and Handel 1964:71).

As geographical distance weakens the extended family, the nuclear family becomes more important. This affects family roles, social life, leisure time, and occupation. "The nuclear family turns inward toward itself, rather than outward toward others, where a member's loyalties would effectively compete with loyalty to spouse and children" (Rainwater and Handel 1964:72).

As husband and wife become more involved with each other and with their children, conjugal roles are less sharply segregated. The husband and wife make joint decisions and cooperate in carrying them out, a situation for which traditional working-class wives have always yearned. Fathers spend their spare time in creative activities around the house and garden, and all the members of the nuclear family join together for recreation. The role of the mother changes from serving the family to participating with it.

The sexual mutuality of the couple increases in the suburbs. A study of family planning revealed that many more of the modern than of the traditional couples believed that sexual relations should be mutually satisfying and reported such relations. The couple has friends in common, instead of separate sets of friends, as in the traditional family, and social relations with these friends sometimes become more important than with relatives. However, the couple does not generally develop interests in the outside world, typical of the middle class, because "such interests are likely to seem . . . harbingers of conjugal segregation in a new guise" (Rainwater and Handel 1964:74, 73).

The typical modern blue-collar family is white, Christian, with two to four children, living in a house in an occupationally mixed suburb. The parents are high-school graduates who have left a lower stratum but have not reached the middle class except in consumer activity. The wife, who worked until the birth of the first child, was generally a clerical or an assembly-line worker. The husband is a factory worker with a steady job and a fairly good income.

In the heterogeneous suburb, the worker may own a house that resembles that of his white-collar neighbor, drive the same kind of car, and dress the same way, but he is faced with many more pressures, and he and his wife are more subject to psychological disorders and marital break-up. Since neither education nor training is responsible for his prosperity, he worries about when he will lose it. He knows that automated machines are replacing workers in many industries and that "guys like him are a dime a dozen." A month's layoff could exhaust all his savings and result in the repossession of his car and appliances or the cashing of insurance policies. He is haunted by the prospect of unemployment, which "is the most frightening, humiliating and angering experience our society has to offer" (AFL-CIO 1963:4).

In the occupationally mixed suburb, the working-class family is not only detached from the security of the extended family, but also from the occupational group, particularly the trade union. "The increased suburban trend will probably accentuate the frequently observed tendency toward diminished union activity and militancy" (Spinrad 1964: 224). Weakened identification with the union probably plays a part in the worker's self-deprecation in the heterogeneous suburb.

The modern blue-collar worker is much more receptive than the traditional worker to "the authority of the media as purveyors of the social, cultural and material goods" (Rainwater and Handel 1964:75). Thus he is much more in debt for many of his possessions, and is often near the margin of financial disaster. This is a source of considerable strain in the family. Yet he makes little effort to upgrade his skills. Whatever energy he has left at the end of the day is conserved for the chores he must do to save money on the maintenance and repair of house and car. "In contrast, many semi-skilled city workers were actively seeking clerical, semi-professional, and small-business positions" (Spinrad 1964:223).

In the heterogeneous suburb both the man and his family are aware of his low status as a factory worker. "The father's job is a point of assessment and evaluation for all family members, particularly in their contacts outside the home" (Dyer 1964:91). If all conditions on the job are favorable—salary, hours of work, type of work, working conditions, fellow workers—the effect of the lower prestige is minimized. But even under the best conditions, blue-collar workers and their families gain less satisfaction from the job than white-collar people.

Although the son in the traditional working-class family frequently follows his father's occupation, the son of the modern worker generally aspires to higher-level employment. The parents do not want their sons to be manual workers or their daughters to marry blue-collar men. However, the father knows "that his children's chances for achieving the good things of life are less than those of the white-collar worker . . . in the community" (Hurvitz 1964:102). This is another source of low self-esteem. Moreover, if his children should advance much beyond his own level, he knows that they will grow apart from him.

The worker's wife has a special problem because she is married to "a man who is not a success by the middle-class standards to which she is exposed and to which she would like to aspire" (Spinrad 1964: 224). She can only "prove her worth as a person by her effectiveness as a mother" and thus she "transfers her loyalty from her husband to her children almost as soon as they appear" (Hurvitz 1964:97). The wife is introduced to middle-class child-rearing values by Spock and other experts, by television programs, the pediatrician, the teacher, and P.T.A. speakers. But the husband's values, which derive from his family and from other working-class men, remain traditional. The "differential value system" in the modern blue-collar family is another source of conflict.

The husband feels he must convey to his children values for survival and advancement in a harsh world full of competing adversaries. He tries to teach his children to be tough and to get ahead because they fear him. He encourages them to be aggressive, threatens and punishes them, and ridicules them for failure. The wife rejects these attitudes in a man who did not himself get ahead, for the successful men are permissive with their children. The husband knows that his own father's authoritarianism did not prepare him for advancement, but permissiveness is an alien philosophy and too difficult to practice.

The children identify with the mother, who is supportive and tries to use "love-oriented" discipline, and the father feels superfluous and rejected in his own family. Aware of his limitations, "the husband does not have a consistent positive model to present . . . and this in turn reinforces his feelings of inadequacy" (Hurvitz 1964:105).

THE URBAN LOWER-WORKING-CLASS FAMILY

Upper-class evaluation of lower-class life appears to have been harsh in all stratified civilizations through the ages. In the United States, the upper and middle classes have applied the same stereotypes to the working classes as to immigrant, racial, and ethnic minorities (Rodman 1964:60). The lower classes are stigmatized particularly because their family life is deemed immoral. The disproportionate numbers of unmarried mothers, deserting fathers and illegitimate children among these classes are viewed by most social scientists as problems arising out of poverty, but a few scholars regard them as solutions to such problems.

In the early 1960s, the lower working class comprised a fourth to a fifth of the population (S. M. Miller 1964a:12); it becomes more numerous during depressions and decreases in times of prosperity. The lower working class lives at or below the poverty line, for about 35 percent of the family heads are not in the labor force. Almost 50 percent of the poor live in urban areas. They are largely older settlers in the slums and refugees from the land, such as Southern mountaineer whites and Southern blacks, Mexican-Americans, and Puerto Ricans (S. M. Miller 1964b:6).

S. M. Miller divides the lower working class into four groupings— the "stable" poor, the "copers," the "strained" and the "unstable"— with considerable intergroup shifting, depending on the degree of economic and family stability.

The stable poor, who have economic and family security, are mainly white. Most are farm, rural nonfarm and small-town persons, but about 30 percent live in metropolitan areas. The children of the stable poor are the most likely to move upward in education and occupation.

Families that remain stable in the face of economic insecurity are the "copers." They become more numerous during layoffs, and include a considerable number of black people. "Children of downwardly mobile families have a better chance of rising occupationally than children of families which have been at this low level for some generations" (S. M. Miller 1964a:16). When low-income families are also strained by the deviant behavior of a family member, their children have fewer chances of rising than those of the "copers."

The traits of the most unstable bottom group are those that are considered typical of "all who are poor or who are manual workers" (S. M. Miller 1964a:23). The "unstable" or "chronic" or "hard-core" poor have neither economic nor family security. They are the newcomers to industrial and urban life, who have not yet developed "the disciplined, structural and traditional approach of the stable worker" (S. M. Miller and Riessman 1964:34). The "hard-core" poor live in a state of crisis and are "constantly trying to make do with string where rope is needed" (S. M. Miller and Riessman 1964:17). They depend more exclusively than any other group on peers, the extended family and neighbors for "both routine services and help in crises that are not so readily available to people in this class from the . . . more impersonal institutions of society" (W. B. Miller 1958:14). At the same time the extended family is often unstable and strife-ridden.

Most of the "hard-core" poor receive welfare assistance which, "in its present form tends to encourage dependence, withdrawal, diffused hostility, indifference, ennui" (S. M. Miller 1964d:302), but they are generally unable to handle dependence and hostility. They have a high incidence of alcoholism, drug addiction, prostitution, venereal disease, broken families, juvenile delinquency, school dropouts, and physical and mental illness.

According to the Midtown Manhattan Study, even when upper and lower classes suffer the same degree of stress in childhood, the personality disorders of the upper classes are less serious. The sick-well ratio in the lowest of the six socioeconomic levels in Manhattan was more than ten times greater than in the highest stratum, and more than three times greater in the lowest than in the highest stratum of manual workers (Srole et al. 1962:31). In a nationwide survey in which the subjects analyzed their own mental health, skilled workers and their wives were found to be the least likely to admit to any worries. Semi-skilled workers, however, were not very happy in general or in their marriages, and their wives frequently reported that they felt they were about to have a nervous breakdown. Unskilled workers were more generally unhappy and had a more negative self-image than any other group. The wives blamed the husbands for their unhappiness, and these wives, too, "feel that they are constantly on the verge of a nervous breakdown" (Gurin, Veroff, and Feld 1960:227).

Cohen and Hodges (1963) describe the lower-working-class family as both patriarchal and mother-centered. When the man is working he receives primary consideration, but he also exempts himself from all household responsibilities, which his wife must assume by default. The husband believes that he should be the boss in "a general and not a functionally circumscribed sense." He has a "compulsive need to affirm, and from time to time to exert, his power in the household," equating "respect for his role as husband and father with *compliance* with his will" (p. 327). When he becomes a parent the lower-blue-collar worker identifies with the harsh authoritarianism of his own father, and he demands respect and obedience from his children. At the same time he is "other directed" and sensitive to the opinions in his milieu, and believes that "one of the most important things that can be taught a child is how to mix well, make friends and be popular" (p. 316).

The lower-working-class man rarely repairs or improves his home even though, with longer stretches of unemployment, he has more free time than men in the other strata. Where the conjugal family is unstable, a greater reluctance to invest heavily in the house might be expected. However, he spends a good deal of money on his car and appliances.

The prevailing market value of the LL's [lower-lower's] car, television, and basic appliances averages almost 20 percent higher than the average value of equivalent upper-blue-collar possessions, despite a median family income that is fully one-third lower (Cohen and Hodges 1963:330).

Since he is almost always subordinate and powerless in the world of work, the lower-blue-collar worker polarizes people into two classes, the strong and the weak, the good and the bad. He condemns more severely than men in the other classes anyone who is deviant—"the atheist, the homosexual, the 'un-American,' the radical, the artist-intellectual" (Cohen and Hodges 1963:321), and the narcotics addict and seller. But above all, he is consistently antagonistic to racial and ethnic minorities.

The problems of the "colored" lower working class, which increasingly comprises the bulk of the poor in metropolitan areas, are greater than those of the white poor because of racial and ethnic discrimination. While the absolute level of income is higher for the urban than the rural colored, the difference in income between white and colored people in the United States is "greater in urban than in rural areas" (Rodman 1968:575). Also, discrimination in housing creates tremendous dissatisfaction with the neighborhood, whereas some white working-class communities are very well integrated, and those who wish to leave a white ghetto may do so much more easily than those in the colored ghetto.

The dissatisfaction resulting from greater deprivation and discrimination has a drastic effect on the family life of the colored poor. Since the family stability of all classes, in the United States and many other countries, is linked to the primary role of the man as breadwinner, the man who cannot support his family is devalued, becomes marginal to the family, and leaves it or is forced out. Many black women, like the women in the San Juan slums, "develop a negative attitude toward men and marriage in general," partly because of their own experiences "and partly as a result of prevalent community attitudes" (Rodman 1968: 758). Goode, however, points out that even where illegitimacy rates are high the majority of people marry, which indicates a general acceptance of dominant values (1946:29).

On the other hand, Walter Miller finds that the values of the lower working class, which directly influence "between 40 and 60 percent of all Americans," regardless of the proportion of the total population which they comprise at any particular period, "constitute a distinctive *patterning* of concerns which differs significantly, both in rank order and weighting, from that of American middle-class culture" (1958: 6–7). The basic form of lower working-class marriage is "serial monogamy," and the female-based household is the primary child-rearing unit. These mores, which violate middle-class norms, are merely a "byproduct of actions oriented to the lower-class system" (1958:19).

The nonlegal marital "solutions of the lower class to the basic occupational-earning problem faced by the man" (Rodman 1968:758) are more fluid than legal marriage and enable men and women to end a relationship more easily. Woman-headed households are "alternative or secondary norms rather than forms of disorganization" (S. M. Miller 1964a:47) for family stability depends on the ability to cope with problems and not solely on the presence of a permanent male head:

the children are being fed, although not necessarily on a schedule; the family meets its obligations, so that it is not forced to keep on the move; children are not getting into much more trouble than other children in the neighborhood (S. M. Miller 1964a:13).

Schwartz and Henderson, however, maintain that the "father-dominated home," in which there is "a relatively high level of reported obedience to fathers" (1964:466) is more stable than the matrifocal family. Jobless black fathers may be well adjusted to a life of unemployment and do not give up their authority role. In fact, lower-class black workers are as authoritarian and traditional as their white counterparts and strongly enforce obedience from their children (Stamler 1964:288–289).

Rodman believes that the broken family and the matrifocal household "are not well adapted to the task of socializing children for achievement in middle-class terms." Children from such families are more likely to be delinquent, and delinquents from broken homes are more likely to be recidivists, the damaging effects being greater for girls and younger children (1968:759). The source of the problem, however, lies in the total social system, not merely in the one institution of the family, for children in segregated schools, even those from patrifocal families, are less likely to achieve than those in integrated schools (Coleman et al. 1966).

Moreover, the family system in which the husband is absent or peripheral is generally defined in negative terms, as a deviant social unit, by Western social scientists. In those areas of the non-Western world, such as Africa and Indonesia, where the mother's role is positively valued and is structurally central, the matrifocal family occurs in a wide range of kinship systems and socioeconomic contexts, for example, among the patrilineal Igbo of Southeast Nigeria (Uchendu 1965), the bilateral Javanese (Geertz 1961), and the matrilineal Adjehnese and Minangkabau of Sumatra (Turner 1971).

The factors which appear to contribute to matrifocality in these cultures are the relative economic, political, and religious equality of women and men, and an emphasis on the mother-child bond (Geertz 1961). Although the mother-child relationship is also emphasized in the West, the subordinate status of women in the major institutions, including the family, leads to the view of the matrifocal family as an aberrant social unit.

Working in a three-year project for the control of gang delinquency, Walter Miller (1958) studied the values of black and white adolescents in twenty-one corner groups in a slum district of a large Eastern city. Miller found that their major goal was "belonging," and while this is also a primary concern of middle-class adolescents, belonging to a peer group is particularly important for a boy brought up only by a mother. The one-sex peer group constitutes "the major psychic force and reference group for those over twelve or thirteen."

In many ways it is the most stable and solidary primary group he has ever belonged to; for boys reared in female-based households the corner group provides the first real opportunity to learn essential aspects of the male role in the context of peers facing similar problems of sex-role identification (1958:14).

These groups sought to attain as quickly as possible the status of adulthood, symbolized by the possession of a car and money; the right to smoke, drink, and gamble; and unrestricted freedom of movement. Because of their intense desire to acquire these symbols, they participated in illegal activities more recklessly than the lower-class adult. To maintain the high level of intragroup solidarity necessary for their activities, the groups excluded disturbed individuals and admitted only those who shared "to an unusually high degree both the *capacity* and *motivation*" to conform to the norms of the milieu. These norms centered around six focal concerns—trouble, toughness, smartness, excitement, fate, and autonomy.

"Getting into trouble" and "staying out of trouble" are major lower-class concerns involving relationships with official authorities. Law-abiding behavior occurs more often from the desire to stay out of trouble than from a commitment to moral values. "Getting into trouble" is a means to several goals: prestige in gangs, excitement or risk, "the covertly valued desire to be 'cared for' and subject to external constraint."

Toughness, manifested by physical prowess, scorn of intellectuality, and the view of women as objects of conquest, is related to a "compulsive reaction-formation" against a childhood in a female-based household in a patriarchal society. Linked to toughness is the concern about homosexuality, which "runs like a persistent thread through lower-class culture." Homosexuality is also related to the "aggressive verbal and physical interaction" which disguises "strongly affectionate feelings toward other men" in the gang. The model for the "tough guy" is the movie or television gangster, cowboy, and private detective.

Smartness is seen as the capacity to achieve goals "through a maximum use of mental agility and a minimum use of physical effort." Corner-group leaders are both tough and smart, but the smart leader has more prestige than the one who is merely tough. The ability to engage in ingenious, aggressive repartee is a component of smartness, and "a very high premium is placed on hair-trigger responsiveness, inventiveness, and the acute exercise of mental faculties." The media model is the professional gambler, the "con man" who outwits others.

Periods of excitement alternate with repetitive routine in the life of many lower-class working people. Excitement is achieved through sex, aggression, drinking, gambling, and music. "Sought risk and desired danger" break up periods of doing nothing in the company of peers.

"Achieving great material rewards, . . . valued in the lower class as well as in other parts of American culture, is a recurrent theme in lower-class fantasy and folk lore," Miller points out. Such rewards are considered to be a matter of fate and luck, and implicit in this view is a sense of the "futility of directed effort towards a goal." Thus gambling is connected with the belief in luck, as well as with toughness, smartness, and excitement.

Autonomy or independence seemingly has the same high value among the lower classes as in the rest of the society. But "the pose of tough rebellious independence often assumed by the lower class person frequently conceals powerful dependence cravings," Miller observes. Authoritarianism and the desire for nurture are closely connected, even while strong resentment is often expressed about unjust or coercive authority. "To be restrictively or firmly controlled is to be cared for," and when lower-class people are released from highly restrictive social environments, like the armed forces, prison, mental hospitals, and reform schools, they often act in such a way as to be recommitted. The behavior of lower-class youngsters in the public schools is frequently a problem because "it generally cannot command the coercive controls implicitly sought" (W. B. Miller 1958:8–15).

Although weighted and ranked differently, many lower-class values are shared by the total society. Most American boys learn to value toughness as a desirable male quality. People who succeed in accumulating wealth, by any means, are considered smart in all social strata, for the gaining of great material rewards is a widely shared fantasy. Aggressive verbal skills are basic to business, political, and social success throughout the United States. The search for excitement is a national theme, as drinking and gambling are national pastimes. The concern about homosexuality "runs like a persistent thread" through all of American culture, and the view of woman as an object of sexual conquest is hardly restricted to the lower classes. A very large number of Americans tend to be biased against the "egg-head," the atheist, the radical, the deviant in behavior and appearance.

However, the loss of faith in the value of work, the belief in fate and luck, extra-legal marital arrangements, great dependency needs, and extreme violence and aggression are more characteristic of the lower working class than of any other social stratum.

The Working-Class World

For approximately three centuries the United States was developed by mobility, both geographical and social, and upward mobility was the primary goal of the American people. As the opportunities for upward mobility became circumscribed with the growth of large-scale business and government, the values of hard work, striving, and individual initiative, the keys to upward mobility, became less important, and alternative values of stability and security became dominant not only for the working classes, but also for large segments of the middle class.

In American society work performs a number of functions. In the Protestant ethic it is the central theme, an end in itself. It is the culturally defined means of making money, which is basic for subsistence as well as for the material goods that bring comfort, enjoyment and prestige. A work-oriented society respects people for the kind of work they do and the amount of money their work brings them, and occupation and income define social classes. Through his work a man ties the world of the family into the social order. Work is also the way to self-realization. "The major activities of the individual must directly satisfy his own creative and emotional impulses, must always be something more than means to an end" (Sapir 1959:92).

For much of the middle and upper classes work performs all or most of these functions, for these classes have the education and professional training that now make possible the achievement of all the social goals. But throughout the blue-collar classes, where economic insecurity is most threatening, the categorical imperative is continuing employment to provide for subsistence. Even the most powerful unions have little or no control over changing social forces such as international trade and world markets, depressions, automation, plant relocation and layoff.

For the upper working class, work provides some of the valued material goods. It anchors the worker and his family in a specific category in society, albeit an inferior one. But it is not generally the means to upward mobility, nor the path to respect and prestige from the society as a whole, nor a source of personal gratification. When the worker denigrates factory work and hopes his children will escape from it, he does not merely share the goal of upward mobility or desire for prestige, but the dominant value that work should be meaningful. Only the skilled craftsmen appear to be unalienated from their work and want their sons to follow their occupations. In the suburbs, the "modern" worker uses his leisure time not for acquiring additional skills that might upgrade him, but for creative activities in the home and garden that are apparently more meaningful.

For the lower working class, work offers few or no satisfactions. Long stretches of unemployment or irregular employment provide neither economic nor family stability, nor an assured place in the social system, nor the valued consumer goods. Thus a large segment of the lower working class devalues work as a means to any goal, and adopts values that are variant in the culture. For some, the major means of achieving goals becomes crime, which is a factor in all social strata, and a sanctified theme in the mass media. Others adopt the values of the culture of unemployment and resist work even when opportunities arise. For these a steady income from a state agency removes many pressures and ensures a more predictable life. On the other hand, living on welfare induces a state of dependency and hostility in a work-oriented culture. Also out of the culture of unemployment emerged the minority movements for racial and ethnic equality and opportunity.

In the face of the economic insecurity that threatens all segments of the blue-collar working class, the worker develops strong drives toward security and stability, which he attempts to achieve through the extended family, peer groups, and the community. But these groups are themselves sources of discord and conflict, especially in their effect on the nuclear family. The nuclear working-class family is heavily burdened. Even the family of the most highly paid skilled worker suffers deprivation during periods of unemployment and is pervaded by anxiety because of indebtedness due to installment buying. The nuclear family bears the brunt of the self-deprecation experienced by family members because of the father's unrespected occupational-earner role. Except in the suburbs, the extended family and peer groups compete strongly and often disruptively with relationships within the nuclear family. The divorce rate rises steadily from "professional" to "craftsman," but increases very sharply in the categories of "service" worker and "laborer" (Goode, 1946:89).

Where the man's present and future occupational status appears to be hopeless and his earning power is most uncertain, not only is the divorce rate the highest, but legal marriage is most frequently by-passed in favor of more fluid relationships that are easier to terminate. In such a situation the matrifocal family emerges. On the one hand, the research indicates that broken families, equated with matrifocal households, have a higher rate of juvenile delinquency, affect girls and younger children most drastically, and prepare children least adequately for academic achievement. On the other hand, family stability seems to depend not on the sex that heads the family, but on a steady income which permits the adequate handling of economic problems and child care. Also, the successful preparation of children for educational achievement seems to depend not on the fact that the family is father-headed, but on racial integration of the schools.

In all segments of the working class, except the modern family in the suburbs, conjugal roles are sharply segregated, and child-rearing values and practices tend to be authoritarian and traditional, especially when compared with the middle class. When compared with Europeans, however, American parents, since the settlement of the nation, have been much less tradition-bound and more tolerant of children's impulses and desires.

The man who was most subject to authoritarianism from his own father and is most subject to economic pressures and insecurity most requires submissiveness and obedience from his wife and children. To the extent that workers exercise some control over their lives, mainly through unions that are democratic, they see the world in less harsh terms and transmit a less forbidding image of society to their children. To the extent that they receive respect from the community or their reference groups, they offer respect to the child. The small group is so essential for the individual that where it is destroyed the individual is atomized and alienated from cultural values (Homans 1950:457).

But the hard-core poor are the least protected by unions, democratic or otherwise. This group is the most powerless vis-à-vis employers and the official agencies, and their children suffer most from authoritarianism. The chronic poor have the least stable reference groups and receive little or no respect from the community, and the child is not respected. Violence and hostility are the least controlled among this segment of the poor, and in the home the children suffer most from aggression. Parents in this group are the most self-rejecting and the most rejecting of their children. The working class as a whole and the lower working class, in particular, are the least tolerant of any kind of deviations, and their mental health is poorest.

As the focal concerns of the working class are differently ordered and weighted than those of the middle class, so is strain "differently patterned on various social levels so that . . . it blends with its cultural setting."

In the case of the socially disintegrated community, culturally distinctive features like a high frequency of violence, crime, and delinquency easily channel the vital strivings of persons under stress, providing a direction for strain to take (Honigmann 1967:414).

It is in the lower working class that the vast majority of Puerto Rican migrants in New York are found.

CHAPTER 10

The Migrants in New York City

The major stresses experienced by the Puerto Rican rural migrants in New York City derive from several causes. They originate partly from American attitudes toward newcomers, partly from problems of Puerto Rican identity, partly from their economic, social, and political difficulties, and partly from the even greater dysfunction of traditional roles in New York than in San Juan, as manifested in conflicts between parents, and between parents and children. But acculturation in New York also brings benefits, and a surprising number of the migrants, especially in the second generation, achieve many of their goals.

Acculturation and Assimilation: Theory and Practice

Acculturation has been defined as comprehending "those phenomena which result when groups of individuals having different cultures come into continuous first hand contact, with subsequent changes in the original culture patterns of either or both groups" (Redfield, Linton, and Herskovitz 1936:149).

In order to identify the problems of acculturating peoples, it is necessary "to determine the depth of commitment to certain shared patterns and values and consequently to assess the difficulties of accepting changes."[1] A crucial factor is the flexibility of the acculturating group. Some people take acculturation in their stride. Others "have a kind of all-or-nothing rigidity," as Felix Keesing (1959:39) expresses it. Most resistant to change are the "characteristics acquired in early personality

[1]Social Science Research Council. Acculturation: An Explanatory Formulation, *American Anthropologist* 56:993.

training, in intimate family customs, in use and enjoyment of staple foods, and, perhaps above all else, in beliefs . . . relating to 'black' magic . . . in areas of life marked by great personal insecurity and fear" (Keesing 1959:398).

Equally important is the flexibility of the host culture in accepting the differences of the acculturating peoples. In the United States the speed and ease with which immigrant groups acculturate also depend "on the degree of native sociocultural congruity" with "the basically Anglo-Saxon, urban, industrial, and Protestant trends that are . . . dominant . . . in the cultural fabric of . . . America" (Srole et al. 1962:288).

Every type of acculturation, but particularly "antagonistic acculturation," is the "outcome of a bilateral challenge resulting from sociocultural contact" (Devereux and Loeb 1943:146). The individual who cannot meet the challenges of either the acculturating or the host system is the " 'marginal man,' a cultural hybrid on the verge of two different patterns of group life, not knowing to which . . . he belongs" (Schuetz 1960:109).

Acculturation is only "the first of the types of assimilation to occur when a minority group arrives on the scene." Acculturation takes place as the newcomer learns the language and behavior patterns of the core culture, but successful acculturation does not necessarily eliminate prejudice and discrimination against the immigrant. Structural assimilation occurs, and all other types of assimilation, including intermarriage, follow only when the acculturating group is admitted "into the social cliques, clubs, and institutions of the core society at the primary group level" (Gordon 1964:77, 81).

Structural assimilation has not taken place to any substantial degree in the United States because of the interacting attitudes of both dominant and minority groups. The American-born citizen has never invited into his primary group life the "hordes of alien newcomers," not to mention the racial minorities. And the immigrant was averse to giving up his own institutions, for the price paid by the ethnic group for structural assimilation is its disappearance "as a separate entity and the evaporation of its distinctive values." Thus the United States is a nation of many and diverse peoples, created by acculturation "without massive structural intermingling" (Gordon 1964:81, 114).

In the course of American immigration three main philosophies of acculturation and assimilation emerged: "Anglo-conformity," the "melting-pot" theory, and "cultural pluralism."

Anglo-conformity, "probably still the dominant implicit theory of assimilation in America, though not unchallenged," assumes that it is eminently desirable to maintain the predominance of the English language, institutions, and cultural patterns in American life, and that newcomers should adapt to these as quickly as possible. In their treatment of the immigrant, Anglo-conformists "flayed his alienness with thinly veiled contempt, ignored his stabilizing ties to the groups which made him a person in the sociological sense, and widened the gap between himself and his children" (Gordon 1964:107, 106).

While immigration is everywhere associated with some stress, it is particularly stressful in the United States.

There is evidence that where . . . a neutral attitude is taken toward the immigrant clinging to his ethnic group, the rates of hospitalization tend to be low. This is the case in Canada. But in countries which advocate a dispersal of the immigrants, adoption of the local language, and rapid transition from traditional customs to the customs of the new country, which discourage immigrants from . . . forming a strong ethnic base, the rate of hospitalization is high. This is the case in Australia and the United States . . . [which] have as a dominant cultural theme . . . individuality which results in hostility or disdain toward those who demonstrate any dependence upon ethnic groups (Fitzpatrick and Gould 1968:138–139).

Although Anglo-conformity had a limited success with the immigrants themselves, it was "overwhelmingly triumphant" with the children of the European immigrants.

The melting-pot theory presumes a merging of all the different cultures in the United States into a distinctive "American way of life." The historian Frederick Jackson Turner regarded the frontier as the biological and cultural melting pot of America, and Israel Zangwill, the playwright, envisaged the cities as the melting pot of all religions and races. But an investigation of intermarriage trends in the 1940s showed that the United States was a triple melting pot, based on religious differences (Kennedy 1944). The three major religions have tended to produce, at different speeds, "products which are culturally very similar, while at the same time they remain structurally separate" (Gordon 1964:131). From an overwhelmingly Protestant nation in the nineteenth century, America has become a country of Protestants, Catholics, and Jews. But because of racial discrimination "the colored" minorities remain outside of the white religious communities.

The immigrants themselves rejected the philosophies of Anglo-conformity and the melting pot. At the beginning of the nineteenth century they began to ask the federal government for land bases of their own, but were always refused. However, they banded together informally and maintained their own languages and institutions. "Cultural pluralism was a fact in American society before it became a theory" (Gordon 1964:135).

The settlement houses in the latter part of the nineteenth century were among the first to defend the ethnic cultures. Throughout the twentieth century many writers have portrayed the life-styles of the different ethnic groups and defended their right to retain their differences. The public schools have been called upon to teach respect for the ethnic cultures and for their contributions to the development of the nation, and to teach the descendants of the immigrants pride in their cultural heritage so that they would have a firm ground on which to stand and would not need to equivocate about their identity.

According to Gordon, however, cultural pluralism is a minor key to the understanding of American society. Although a number of individual immigrants or their children have been extremely influential in American life, "the impact of minority group culture has been of modest dimensions . . . in most areas, and significantly extensive in only one —the area of institutional religion." The dominant social condition is structural pluralism—"a structural separation on the basis of race and religion" (1964:109, 235).

An early exponent of the view that the poor should break through this condition of structural pluralism in order to gain equal access to the social institutions was Saul Alinsky. He advocated that the poor transcend ethnic, racial, and religious differences and organize in power blocs around issues generating conflict with the established power structure, not only to further their common interests but also to help them shake off the apathy of slum life. Alinsky adapted the organizational tactics of the industrial union organizers because of the similar conditions of the slum-dweller and the unorganized factory worker (Anderson 1966). "The laborer's perception of himself has improved in direct ratio as his union has earned respect for itself as a power structure in the community" (Dodson 1968:43).

In the past the white ethnic youth who learned the language, manners, and dress of the core society and subscribed to the dominant myths and rituals was given a little piece of the pie. Most Americans, therefore, never had to learn to respect differences, for many of the most capable people alienated themselves from their ethnic groups in order to escape the harsh conditions of the slums and advance in American society. "Thus we have always siphoned off the potential leadership of the minority and left the group to stew in its own problems. We have, as a consequence, never solved the problem of the slums" (Dodson 1968:92). However, the black and the colored Spanish-speaking youth cannot escape their identity and therefore cannot escape the effects of prejudice. When the slum-dweller has no hope of obtaining a better life either for himself or for his children, "there is disengagement from the mythologies of the dominant group." When disengagement is accompanied by restlessness, "a little more welfare is squirted on people to keep them tranquilized," for "the powerful have always found it easier to provide welfare services . . . than share power" with groups that are powerless (Dodson 1968:28).

Moreover, with the erosion of ethnic differences by mass culture, the individual now views his group in terms of its power status. When the ethnic group is powerless, the individual becomes either overly aggressive or apathetic. But if the group integrates into the larger society by economic, political, and social action, the capable person becomes a leader in his own community and no longer needs to adjust his personality to the dominant patterns.

There is evidence of increasing collaboration among the poor across racial, ethnic, and religious lines, but the barriers between the groups are still strong as they fight one another for jobs in a contracting economy.

New York, the City of Immigrants

The rural migrant who lives in a shantytown in San Juan preserves his folk culture for a time and urbanizes gradually. But in New York he must adapt quickly to one of the most highly urbanized cities in the world, in a different culture, with a different language and climate.

New York is "the world's supreme metropolis" (Srole et al. 1962: 102). It is the place where men feel "their lives will gloriously be fulfilled and their hunger fed" (Wolfe 1939:229). It draws to itself "the restless, the dissatisfied and the ambitious, who have demanded more from life than the circumstances of their birth offered them" (Waugh 1956).

The metropolis is preeminently the place offering opportunities for economic and social advancement. In drawing to itself a migrant population largely motivated to actualize these opportunities, a hypercompetitive society is created of people . . . who . . . must hurry even to remain where they are (Srole et al. 1962:117).

New York took on its heterogeneous character at birth. Already by 1660 "eighteen languages were spoken . . . at the tip of Manhattan Island" (Glazer and Moynihan 1963:1). The various ethnic groups that came with resources or skills had few problems adjusting to the city, but the poor, unskilled laborer had little opportunity until New York became an industrial center in the nineteenth century. The growing number of unskilled gave rise to increasing complaints about pauperism and delinquency, and by 1824 the demand for greater police action was established as a permanent metropolitan pattern.

Yet the economic development of the city depended on continuing immigration. From earliest times the Yankees migrated from New England to New York. When New York State abolished slavery in 1827, many free blacks and fugitive slaves came to the city, worked in the service trades, and led a coherent communal life centered around their churches. Although their schools were segregated and they had other grievances, their burdens were lighter than those of blacks in other parts of the country. From 1820 to 1840 the main European immigrants were English, French, and German who came with money and skills, and became part of the artisan groups in the city. The great potato famines in the middle of the nineteenth century led to the influx of the starving peasants of Ireland and Germany.

From the outset, housing could not keep pace with immigration. The newcomers had to take the cheapest accommodations in old commercial and residential buildings that had been converted into multiple-family dwellings. Rented on a weekly basis, these provided the landlords a much higher income than more respectable property. Since the buildings were rarely repaired and soon deteriorated, a housing shortage was created which became another permanent feature of the city. At about mid-century, the walk-up tenements were more crowded than slum dwellings in almost any other city in the world.

As pleasant residential areas became overpopulated, the earlier, more prosperous residents moved to the outskirts of the city. "In addition on the outskirts . . . were shanty settlements where squatters without legal title made their homes" (Handlin 1959:16). In 1860 the Germans had a shantytown on the East River and the Irish, on the Hudson.

As the population grew, so did disease, the foreign-born always being the most numerous victims. Organized gambling and policy games were a major problem before 1850, with the Irish disproportionately involved in both crime and pauperism. Occasionally the Irish, Germans, and blacks fought each other. The rise in disease, pauperism, and crime led to outbreaks of open hostility against the immigrants from the 1830s onward, which partly expressed native resentment against economic competition from the newcomers. But although anti-immigrant movements tried to limit political rights, particularly of the Irish Catholics, they did not restrict immigration.

Under such circumstances people of common background formed tightly knit groups and established their own churches, newspapers, theaters, militias, fire companies, and mutual aid and fraternal societies, which functioned in banking, insurance, and building and loan associations. Most people accepted the dominant middle-class values.

Even the mass of former peasants, who could not in their own lives apply the American axioms of thrift, hard work, advancement and progress, recognized that these were the keys to respect and status in the United States (Handlin 1959:18).

After 1870 New York became a great industrial and financial metropolis, and by the beginning of the twentieth century it was the most important seaport in the nation. It continued to grow by migration from other parts of the country and, even more, by immigration from Europe. The Scandinavians joined the continuing stream of Irish and German immigrants, and after 1880 there was mounting emigration of landless peasants from Sicily and southern Italy, Greece, Rumania, the Slavic and Baltic countries, and of Jews from Russia and the Austrian Empire.

Economic information was now more widely disseminated, and the volume of immigration corresponded more closely with the fluctuations of the business cycle. Since transportation within the United States had improved, the later immigrants went to other cities besides New York. Nevertheless, as Handlin points out, in 1890 the foreign-born and their children constituted about 80 percent of the population of Manhattan. The continuously rising complaints about the concentration of immigrants in New York "really reflected dissatisfaction with the effects of industrialization and focused upon the immigrants as symbols of a change other Americans could not control" (1959:23).

The immigrants resisted both government and private attempts to redistribute them to the interior because they wanted to live in the ethnic enclaves that were already established in the cities.

The efforts to move the immigrants into agriculture ran contrary to the dominant tendencies of the American economy at the end of the nineteenth century. The sons of native farmers were themselves deserting their homestead to move to the cities, and the immigrants felt the same attraction (Handlin 1959:23).

The later immigrants also found it easier to earn a living because the manufacturing, construction, and building trades were expanding and required abundant cheap labor. The vast majority, being unskilled and poor, were always compelled to take the jobs with the lowest pay and the most difficult working conditions, which were abandoned by older residents as soon as possible. But as discrimination against the newer arrivals increased after the turn of the century, escape from the ranks of unskilled labor became more difficult, even for the second generation. Nevertheless, the immigrants were able to advance through petty trade, peddling, contracting, the service trades, the professions, the stage and athletics, and gambling and other illegal activities. The influence of middle-class leadership militated against the growth of a strong trade-union movement, and after 1915 manpower shortages and hostility to unions helped create labor racketeers (Handlin 1959:26).

With the support of the ethnic group, the second generation found employment in government, entered the professions and, to some extent, the church, where they "were sometimes better off than the children of the natives." For most New Yorkers ethnic affiliations remained strong beyond the third generation. "Children who grew up within the same environment tended to marry within the group so that the ethnic ties passed from generation to generation" (Handlin 1959:25, 28). The Jews rose exceptionally fast and the Irish, exceptionally slowly, because of differences in their European experience and in ethnic values about thrift and education.

Those who accepted the public school not only acquired valuable skills from it, but also values which stressed the importance of the climb upward. For such there were more opportunities to penetrate into the professional and managerial ranks than were open to their contemporaries who either left the school early or were segregated in ethnic parochial schools (Handlin 1959:27).

The descendants of the English were found mainly in the middle and upper classes. The less wealthy among them identified upward mobility with good family, neighborhood, church, school, and social group, and the wrong identifications could create obstacles. That anxiety was the dynamic element in their situation, so that they felt compelled to move at the first sign of a new ethnic group in their neighborhood. After 1900, the subway brought many outlying regions within cheap and easy access to the city, and "the one-family house and garden . . . became a symbol of their Americanism" (Handlin 1959:30).

The second generation in each ethnic group imitated the Anglo-American way of life, and also avoided identification with the newer immigrants.

They, and each successive group after them, found themselves drawn into a pattern of Americanization that demanded of them a complex of culture changes in habits and tastes, in family size and language, and also in standards of housing (Handlin 1959:32).

When the later immigrants arrived—particularly the Jews and the Italians—the Irish and Germans, now mainly in the upper blue collar and lower middle classes, competed with the old Americans for better living space. Despite endless experiment the problem of finding decent working-class housing was never solved. This greatly aggravated the difficulties of quickly moving into a limited area a very large number of people who were inexperienced in urban living and unfamiliar with American values. In addition, government in New York was slow to change from a rural pattern and did not adequately protect residents against the disorderliness which helped to produce a pervasive criminality. Although the degree of maladjustment was to some extent determined by pervious cultural background, all those whose situation was precarious were disoriented. The situation of the second generation was also always exceptionally trying because of the difficulty of reconciling dominant values with those of the ethnic group.

The very heterogeneity of New York demanded an accommodation, however, and the multiplicity of groups prevented their isolation in any one sector. As a result, New Yorkers came to feel a sense of pride in the cosmopolitan character of their city, and the diversity came to be regarded as a source of strength. Politics provided a means of adjustment rather than becoming a source of conflict, as in many other cities. New York politicians had to gain the support of a number of groups, and the local political clubs reflected the composition of the mixed neighborhood.

After 1870 voluntary ethnic associations became even more numerous and important, and eased many of the problems of inter-group adjustment. The church was a cohesive social and religious institution. The theater and the press became vital instruments of ethnic expression. Effectively functioning communities helped those with problems and relieved the state of part of the burden of welfare work. They also helped to orient new arrivals to American values (Handlin 1959:38–39).

The ethnic community supplied its members with . . . a pattern of acceptable forms of action and of expression, connected with the forms of the larger society about them, but integrated in a context intelligible in their own lives (Handlin 1959:40).

In all groups those who succeeded in "American" terms became leaders and models for the others and their ability to succeed testified to the possibility of adjustment by the whole group.

During World War I the city remained comparatively untouched by the "red scare" in the rest of the country, for the "tradition of cosmopolitanism preserved New York from the disorder of group conflict." The German-Americans were rarely abused, and the xenophobia that ended immigration was largely absent in New York. "The foreigners had not antagonized the people who lived with them; but they had earned the hostility of the rural folk of the west and the south who had little direct contact with the urban population" (Handlin 1959:41).

The barriers to European immigration during and after World War I resulted in a shortage of unskilled labor in the North and thousands of Southern blacks flocked to the city. This inflow decreased during the depression of the 1930s, but it was resumed during and after World War II, together with mass migrations from Puerto Rico. Today New York is the city with the largest black and Puerto Rican populations in the world.

Most of the new minorities came to New York when public housing was replacing many dilapidated tenements, and when a wide range of new public services was being instituted. But automation was also beginning to eliminate the unskilled jobs by which the earlier immigrants had gained their toehold, and factory wages were beginning to decline.

To solve their economic problems, blacks and Puerto Ricans are increasingly entering the political arena. The political patterns of the city "strengthen the roles of ethnic groups," for the "balanced ticket and the balanced distribution of patronage along ethnic lines have assumed an almost fervid sanctity." However, "class interests and geographical locations are the dominant influences in voting behavior whatever the ethnic group involved" (Glazer and Moynihan 1963:305, 310).

The Puerto Ricans are separated from the Catholics as well as from the blacks by color and culture. But more and more black and Puerto Rican leaders are attempting to transcend ethnic differences and conflicts by common action toward common goals.

Incentives to Puerto Rican Migration

The Puerto Rican migrants who came to New York before World War II were mainly skilled and semiskilled urban workers who were better educated, more regularly employed and better paid than the average on the island (Mills, Senior and Goldsen 1950:25). However, "many, if not most of those who emigrated in the 1950s had never lived in cities and large towns" (Hernández-Alvarez 1967:4).

The composition of the Puerto Rican migration stream varies with changing socioeconomic conditions both on the island and on the mainland. The predominant factor in the prewar period was the pull of New York on people with some skills in an area that had low living standards and a high unemployment rate. When Puerto Rico began to industrialize and agriculture began to decline, migration had less to offer skilled and semiskilled urban dwellers, but a great deal to offer farm workers. Virtually excluded from the prewar migrations because of limited job opportunities for the unskilled and the high cost of transportation, farm workers had much to gain from the postwar opportunities for unskilled labor on the mainland, especially after transportation rates were lowered. The rising level of education in Puerto Rico in the 1950s also better equipped the farm worker for job competition, and employment on the mainland increased his skills.

Migration from a less-developed to a highly-industrialized area is in effect a training experience which contributes to the life-time income of the migrant whether . . . in the new location or . . . the area of origin (Gray 1962:1).

A most important incentive to migration was the large income differential between agricultural and nonagricultural work. "The occupation with the greatest differential in percentage terms through the 1950's was the farm laborers" (Friedlander 1965:117), who, unemployed for several months of the year, derived the maximum income gain from a job in manufacturing or trade in New York:

the rural farm workers, usually being the poorest and least informed, would be the last segment of the population to migrate; but because of the economic advantages that migration offers them, they eventually dominate the composition of the migration stream (Friedlander 1965:114).

From a social point of view, "migration was one form of emancipation from the semi-feudal system of social organization which had rigidly governed the destiny of most Puerto Ricans for centuries" (Hernández-Alvarez 1967:4).

The Problem of Puerto Rican Identity

The earlier immigrants to New York deliberately sought to preserve their traditional cultures, which were rooted in religion or nationality, or both, and they acculturated from a strong sense of ethnic identity. But the Puerto Ricans lack a strong sense of identity, even on the island. The native Indian culture was largely obliterated and Puerto Rican blacks preserved little of their African heritage. Under Spain the vast majority of Puerto Ricans were kept in a state of ignorance and illiteracy and were isolated from the dominant Spanish culture. And unlike the Mexicans, Puerto Ricans were not united in a great revolutionary struggle against Spain. "In Mexico even the poorest slum dwellers have a much richer sense of the past and a deeper identification with Mexican tradition than do Puerto Ricans with their tradition" (O. Lewis 1965:xvii).

The religious experience of the Puerto Rican lower classes has been ambiguous. The gulf between Catholicism and the *jíbaro* is of long standing, and Puerto Rico had no indigenous clergy either under Spain or the United States.

> They did not have that penetrating sense of Catholic identity which comes from a deeply rooted and untroubled folk attachment to Catholicism. . . . Nor did many have a mature conscious loyalty to the Church as an organization. . . . As a result, the sense of identity which was the basis around which ethnic loyalties crystallized in the lives of other immigrants, was weak in the Puerto Ricans before they came (Fitzpatrick 1968:11).

The "Americanization" of Puerto Rico was abrupt and painful. "The social and cultural adjustments to industrialization are evident everywhere, and the distress associated with them is deeply and widely felt. . . . From many points of view, Puerto Ricans have been culturally uprooted before they leave the island" (Fitzpatrick 1968:10). Puerto Rico is neither an American state nor independent, neither fully a member of the North American culture area nor of the Caribbean. The result is "a certain amount of cultural schizophrenia" (Glazer and Moynihan 1963:129).

The tightly knit neighborhoods of the earlier immigrants helped them preserve their ethnic identity and gave strength and support to newcomers as they adjusted to the city. But after World War II, slum clearance in New York destroyed ethnic communities, and the integration policy of public housing interfered with the formation of strong community bases. Because of the shortage of inexpensive housing, Puerto Ricans are dispersed throughout the metropolitan area.

In many ways the Migration Division of the Commonwealth Labor Department in New York City takes the place of the ethnic community. It helps to orient newcomers, tries to obtain jobs for them, and has persuaded many migrants to move to other cities. It is a government agency, however, and not a self-help organization.

> It may very well be that it is because the Puerto Rican group has been so well supplied with paternalistic guidance from their own government, as well as with social services by the city and private agencies, that it has not developed powerful grass-roots organizations (Glazer and Moynihan 1963:110).

Puerto Rico itself may also fulfill the functions of the ethnic community. Low-cost transportation rates enable mainland Puerto Ricans to go back to the island for vacations, for help from family and friends, and to return permanently when life in New York becomes too difficult. But this may prevent identification with either Puerto Rico or the mainland, and may hinder acculturation to the mainland. Return to Europe, on the other hand, was so costly that few of the earlier immigrants could consider repatriation as a solution to their problems.

At the same time as they learned to speak English, the immigrants from the non-English-speaking countries of Europe continued to speak their own language, and this helped them to retain their ethnic identity. But the Spanish language became a source of identity for Puerto Rico only when the United States imposed the learning of English upon its educational system (Steward 1956:500). In the absence of other sources, the Spanish language is regarded as the major and perhaps the only source of Puerto Rican identity. Certainly New York has responded, as it never did for the earlier immigrants, with many kinds of innovations in Spanish, including bilingual programs in the public schools. "There are signs in Spanish in the New York subways and in other places where Puerto Ricans congregate. . . . Thousands of teachers, public servants, clergy, have learned Spanish in order to communicate" (Fitzpatrick 1966:107). Language, however, shares the ambiguity that characterizes all aspects of Puerto Rican identity, for it is intimately associated with ambivalent attitudes toward race and color. Some Puerto Ricans deny their origins by refusing to speak Spanish. Others try to establish *Hispano* credentials by speaking only Spanish.

While racial discrimination prevails in Puerto Rico, Latin Americans view race differently from North Americans. In the United States, people are categorized as either white or black, and "one drop of Negro blood" makes them black, regardless of appearances to the contrary. For Puerto Ricans, however, physical appearance is the criterion for racial identity. They recognize three racial categories—white, black, and intermediate—and most nonwhite Puerto Ricans place themselves in the intermediate category. Moreover, a mulatto, and even a Negro, who is wealthy or politically prominent in Puerto Rico is considered to be socially white. But Americans ascribe "a mixed racial ancestry to all Puerto Ricans . . . [and] racial mixture is equivalent to a Negro social identity" in the United States. The Puerto Rican on the mainland suffers from an identity problem because of "the vicissitudes in the communication and interaction processes which a dissimilar codification of racial criteria creates between Puerto Ricans and North Americans" (Seda-Bonilla 1966:109, 112). This problem is associated with the Spanish language.

Seda-Bonilla found that a group of lower-class Puerto Rican families considered their Yorkville community to be desirable because it excluded Puerto Ricans and blacks. These families hid their origins and "they said they never spoke Spanish in public." In a neighborhood in East Harlem, "second-generation white children . . . also refused to be identified as Puerto Ricans and pretended not to understand Spanish. . . . [Puerto Rican] children were also antagonistic to their parents whom they blamed for the difficulties they had to live through because of their national identity." For some white lower-class Puerto Ricans, "Puerto Ricanness . . . spells out a nonwhite social identity, and when pressed, they often take refuge in 'Spanish' credentials" and refer to themselves as *Hispanos* (Seda-Bonilla 1966:113–114).

A Puerto Rican in the intermediate group is residentially segregated, "finds that he can hold only certain jobs, mix socially only with certain people." He is the true marginal man. "The intermediately colored are the least adapted of all the racial groups. . . . They are not accepted by the American whites and they are reluctant to enter the American Negro community." Although proficiency in English is the most important aspect of acculturation in the United States, the intermediately colored Puerto Rican is reluctant to speak English in public because "he is even more likely to lose the slight advantage he holds in New York over the American Negro." Thus he generally speaks Spanish "so that he will be identified . . . as a Latin . . . for somehow a non-American Negro receives privileged treatment in the New York Community" (Mills, Senior, and Goldsen 1950:133, 154, 134).

According to Seda-Bonilla, black Puerto Ricans in East Harlem find open acceptance in the American black society with credentials of "West Indian." They "also spoke Spanish with ease and showed no anxiety about their Puerto Rican identity." But "the heroes which they selected . . . were American Negroes of outstanding achievement" (1966:115). Chenault, on the other hand, maintained that the American black tended to resent all West Indians, including Puerto Ricans, because they were competitors in the labor market. Chenault also said that "the darker the person from the West Indies is, the more intense his desire to speak only Spanish, and to do so in a louder voice" (1938:150–51).

Language is also one of the barriers between the recent migrants and Puerto Ricans who are long-time residents of New York. Acculturated Puerto Ricans are proud that they can speak English without an accent and are embarrassed by the migrant who generally speaks an accented English or no English at all (Padilla 1958:96).

Second-generation Puerto Ricans generally speak English in the presence of non-Puerto Ricans, and they are offended when they are addressed in Spanish, especially by Americans who assume they cannot speak English. But when English-speaking persons of higher social or economic status patronize Puerto Ricans, they may speak Spanish to express their resentment. For many Puerto Ricans brought up in New York, knowledge of Spanish is no special accomplishment:

> they regard the constant use of Spanish, as well as any other form of behavior that distinguishes them from Americans, as detrimental. . . . Yet, . . . they find themselves having constantly to strive toward maintaining their identification, for in terms of the larger community, they are not Americans (Padilla 1958:100).

The people who call themselves *Indigenistas,* on the other hand, are not filled with self-hate or alienated from their group. "They carry the Puerto Rican credentials of identity with dignity and self assurance. . . . Many individuals . . . even in the third generation spoke Spanish well and exhibited pride in their Puerto Rican origin" (Seda-Bonilla 1966:115). The *Indigenistas* are often leaders in *Aspira* and similar organizations which work "for the defense of Puerto Rican migrants," and for a strong Puerto Rican community which will integrate with the larger society. This group identifies with "the Jews or Italians of forty years ago, rather than with the Negroes of today."

> [It] clearly sees Puerto Ricans as following in the path of the earlier ethnic groups that preceded it, and speaks of them as models of emulation rather than as targets for attack. . . . It has a rather hopeful outlook which emphasizes the group's potential for achievement more than the prejudice and discrimination it meets (Glazer and Moynihan 1963:128).

Since most of the factors which strengthened the identity of the earlier immigrants are absent in the Puerto Rican community, it may be forced to use political power as "a source of cohesion as well as a means of control of its destiny" (Fitzpatrick 1969:66).

Occupations, Income, and Consumer Practices

About 70 percent of the migrants on the mainland live in New York City, which had a Puerto Rican population of about 975,000 in 1968.[2] The great majority are unskilled farm workers, whose "adjustment to urban living will most likely be more difficult than migrants from urban areas" (Macisco 1968:25). In 1964 their median age was 21.7 years, compared with 26.5 for nonwhites and 38.4 for whites.[3]

---

[2]*The New York Times,* November 14, 1968, p. 41.

[3]U. S. Department of Labor, *Labor Force Experience of the Puerto Rican Worker.* Regional Report No. 9. New York: U. S. Department of Labor, Bureau of Labor Statistics, June, 1968, pp. 4–5.

According to the 1960 census, 40 percent of the males and 66 percent of the females were semiskilled operatives; about 18 percent of the men were service workers; about 7 percent of the men and almost 9 percent of the women were clerical and sales workers; and 2.2 percent of the men and 3.8 percent of the women were professional and technical workers (Macisco 1968:27). Like the earlier immigrants, the majority have the jobs that others don't want.

Puerto Ricans use some avenues of mobility which are traditional both on the island and the mainland. Like the island *jíbaro,* migrants move out of the ranks of labor in New York by opening little *bodegas* that cater to distinctive Puerto Rican tastes. But blue-collar workers now find that opening a store requires increased capital, and negotiating loans is very difficult because of "persistent stereotypes among bankers of what constitutes a good risk" (Handlin 1959:75). More and more the chain stores put small and new businesses at a disadvantage. In addition, "the destruction of Puerto Rican businesses in East Harlem, . . . which has been almost entirely leveled for new housing projects, was prodigious" (Glazer and Moynihan 1963:75). Nevertheless, "in the face of heavy competition and a high rate of small business mortality, the New York Puerto Ricans have shown themselves amazingly fertile in spawning small stores" (Glazer and Moynihan 1963:112).

Highly prized routes to upward mobility are those depending on individual talent. After each wave of immigration, "the immigrant needed to accelerate the process of integration, of proving his individual worth, of achieving self-esteem as quickly as possible" (Golden 1958:127). A limited number of Puerto Ricans also move upward through "policy and other forms of gambling, and through rackets associated with narcotics, vice, unions, and business" (Handlin 1959:71). But "there are indications . . . that nepotism . . . among the more successful rackets" (Senior 1961:96) bars most of the migrants:

one of the few distinctions so far between the Puerto Ricans and the early immigrant groups . . . is that the Puerto Ricans have developed no criminal gangs of adults as the Irish, Jews, and Italians did. . . . Many old-time observers in the city believe this lack of an adult underworld is one of the reasons why Puerto Ricans have not yet achieved any power in politics (Wakefield 1959:128).

Since almost nine out of every ten New York Puerto Ricans over age twenty-five have not finished high school, the first generation generally remains in the lower blue-collar class. Moreover, their unemployment rate is high because the "substantial loss of factory jobs here in recent years [is in] the very industrial area in which Puerto Ricans were so heavily concentrated" (Mooney 1968:94), for "all but the lightest forms of factory production have retreated to outlying areas" (Srole et al. 1962:71).

One out of every three Puerto Rican workers living in three of the city's main poverty areas is unemployed, badly underemployed or earning substantially less than a minimum wage. . . . For every officially counted unemployed Puerto Rican worker there are at least two others who have a very real problem in terms of labor force maladjustment. . . . Even among persons living in the city's poverty areas, Puerto Ricans find themselves close to the bottom (Lissner 1968:29).

With the poverty level at $4,000 for a family of four in 1967, the median income of Puerto Ricans in Manhattan was about $3,460, compared with the general Manhattan median of about $5,340 (Grossman 1967:7). The disparity in earnings is due to the fact that the migrants are clustered in the least rewarding occupations rather than to differences in pay rate for a given job. Unlike the earlier immigrants, Puerto Ricans are protected, to a considerable extent, by fair employment practices, minimum wage laws, and unions. About 55 percent of Puerto Rican men and 60 percent of the women in the labor force are union members.

Old timers in the labor movement report that the rise of Puerto Rican leadership in local unions is unusually rapid for a group of recent arrivals. For many, union activity has been the road to political activity (Senior 1968:75).

Since their socioeconomic status is so unfavorable, the Puerto Ricans look to government for help in surviving. About one-seventh of all Puerto Ricans are on public assistance, and they "contribute one-half of the home-relief cases and one-third of the aid-to-dependent children cases" (Glazer and Moynihan 1963:118).

Although a woman without a husband is not ashamed to receive welfare aid, Puerto Rican culture prescribes that men reciprocate free gifts or services. "Only a sick man can justify receiving welfare aid, and in many cases the man claims that his wife is the one who receives it, or that it is for the children" (Padilla 1958:258). Receiving welfare creates problems. Antagonistic neighbors may report an individual who is "making money" from home relief. The caseworker must be informed of other sources of income, which discourages upward mobility. Authority shifts from the father to the caseworker, who plans the family budget.

According to Horwitz, however, Puerto Ricans see welfare only as a source of money, nothing else, and pay little attention to the caseworker.

They used welfare as an economic stabilizer, a guaranteed income in case low-paying restaurant, hotel, nursing-home, hospital, garment-industry jobs could not support a family, or if the exorbitant rents . . . ate up the take-home pay (Horwitz 1969:22).

In 1966 New York City broke the code of silence which prevailed throughout the country about the right to public assistance. The welfare commissioner revealed the extent of poverty in the city and accepted many more applications for home relief and aid to dependent children. In addition, the poor were learning to fight for their welfare rights, so that "the rising case load would bring a crisis in the welfare system and force the nation to adopt some such alternative as the negative income tax or guaranteed annual income" (Horwitz 1969:22).

In 1967, New York City paid "100 percent of the budget deficit—an average of $278 a month for a family of four, including rent," compared with $55 in Mississippi, and $24.50 in Puerto Rico (Kihss 1968b:28). The City Club of New York attributed the 50 percent rise in the city's welfare rolls from 1965 to December, 1967, to

the reluctance of poor people to take low-paying jobs, a growing knowledge of the availability of relief, welfare becoming "a fully accepted part of the poor people's culture," a bureaucracy benefitting from the growth of relief and "a severe breakdown of family life and male responsibility," as well as migration (Kihss 1968b:28).

About 65 percent of welfare assistance in New York is aid to dependent children, largely children denied, abandoned, or deserted by their fathers. The children, "the most tragic group among welfare recipients, become adults before they ever have a childhood."

They suffer a grade retardation twice as great as non-welfare school children. . . . They see adults as enemies. . . . The kids grow up on welfare with the attitude that everything should be free and easy. With parents that work, the kids are different . . . they see things ahead for them (Kihss 1968b:28).

The installment buying practices of low-income Puerto Ricans in New York characterize the entire working class, as well as much of the middle class, both on the island and the mainland. But the rural migrants have no knowledge of the legitimate buying patterns of urban bureaucratic society, and they become involved with a local marketing system which intensifies their economic insecurity.

In 1960, the Bureau of Applied Social Research of Columbia University studied the buying practices of 464 families living in four low-income housing projects in Manhattan. According to Caplovitz, the study was done on behalf of "three New York City settlement houses that had become quite alarmed by the installment debts besetting their neighbors" (1964:111). The population was 45 percent Puerto Rican, 30 percent black and 25 percent white, and 83 percent of the total were migrants from the South and from Puerto Rico. More than 40 percent of the family heads had only an elementary school education, most had unskilled or semiskilled jobs with a median income of about $3,300, and about 15 percent received welfare assistance.

With the least possibility of upward mobility, these families turned to compensatory consumption "as the one sphere in which they can make some progress toward the American dream of success," Caplovitz writes. They bought major durable goods at high prices from the same type of "customer peddlers" who had served immigrants several generations before, and from local stores that advertised "easy credit" plans. The stores established friendly relationships with customers by omitting service charges when payments were late, but their markup was therefore much higher than in department stores. "The most active consumers, those who rely most on credit, and those who experience the most consumer problems tend to be the Puerto Ricans and Negroes, the relatively large . . . and young families" (1964:110, 115).

More than 60 percent of the families had outstanding consumer debts, with no savings to back them up. The heavy credit obligations reached crisis proportions when illness or unemployment suddenly reduced their income. When they missed payments, they suffered legal pressures, their goods were repossessed, they were threatened with garnishments or their salaries were garnisheed, and as a result many were fired. A number of families had bought reconditioned merchandise represented as new, and others were tricked into making purchases by salesmen pretending to be housing authority representatives.

To preserve their goodwill in the neighborhood many merchants used informal personal controls rather than legal pressures. They sent salesmen to visit the families at home, both to collect payments and to sell additional merchandise, or encouraged weekly payment plans to bring customers back into the store for additional purchases. The families were continuously in debt to the merchant in a pattern that recalls the relationship between the sharecropper and the company store. But these unethical and illegal practices persisted because they performed important social functions.

In a society in which consumption is not only a matter of obtaining material conveniences, but also a means of gaining self-respect and winning the respect of others, this marketing system makes consumers of people who fail to meet the requirements of the more legitimate economy. Even the welfare family is able to consume in much the same manner (Caplovitz 1964:117).

Housing and Neighborhood Life

New York is "a very important element in the hopes and dreams of
the islanders for a better life." Puerto Ricans are familiar with many
aspects of life in New York before they arrive and consider it "a
Puerto Rican frontier and not a foreign place" (Padilla 1958:24). The
marked contrast between the rural areas of the island and the American
metropolis, however, makes the Puerto Rican a foreigner, both culturally and psychologically. To the newcomer, faced by the overwhelming number of different worlds in New York, the city appears enormous,
confusing, and chaotic. And the migrants who have been coming to
New York since World War II are confronted not only by the normal
chaos of the city, but also by a desperate housing shortage.

Between 1945 and 1955 slum clearance in New York created "an
enforced population displacement completely unlike any previous population movement in the city's history" (Handlin 1959:85). More than
a third of those who were forced to move were black and Puerto Rican,
and fewer than a third of the movers were relocated in public housing
projects, although the displaced were legally entitled to relocation. The
rest had to find housing as best they could, and the search was always
complicated by the factor of color.

The shock of discovering the significance of discrimination on the mainland
created a marked temptation among the whites to sever their ties with the
group. Many seized whatever opportunity they could to move away to neighborhoods where they would not be known as Puerto Ricans. The colored,
on the other hand, stressed their identification with the group as a means
of keeping themselves apart from the Negroes (Handlin 1959:95).

East Harlem, El Barrio, was the first major settlement of Puerto
Ricans in New York, as it had been for earlier immigrants. But by
1960 slum clearance and housing projects had broken up "the Puerto
Rican concentrations (in the oldest and most decrepit housing, of
course) as soon as they were formed, and prevented new concentrations
from forming" (Glazer and Moynihan 1963:94).

In many sections of the city, public housing "tore down diversity"
and put up a "high-rise ghetto," which resulted in the "hurried relocation of thousands of families . . . and the frantic struggles by former
residents to secure an apartment in the new projects" (Sexton 1965:39).

Relocation has become the symbol of inadequacy and frustration. Relocation
has meant the uprooting of families, enforced homelessness, sacrifice of
neighborhood values, threats to sources of political power, and equally im-

portant, the superimposing of a way of life often inconsistent with the very objective the plan is intended to serve (Meltzer 1953:451).

Public housing barred all those who earned more than a minimum amount, and moved out families when their incomes rose, contributing to the flight of the white middle class from the city. A third of the families in the projects are fatherless, and more than 15 percent are physically or mentally ill. The young people outnumber the adults, and the "youth culture" is very powerful.

Many professionals, including social workers and architects, were disappointed when public housing did not solve all the social and personal problems of the poor. Jane Jacobs, for example, is quoted by Sexton: "There is nothing wrong with these buildings except that, humanly speaking, they stink. Sanitary steam-heated apartments are no substitute for warm-hearted neighbors, even if they live in verminous cold-water flats." According to Sexton, however, "The poor don't seem to agree. They clearly prefer sanitation and steam heat to warm-hearted neighbors, though they would like to have both. . . . For the poor, the villain is more often the slumlord" (1965:42).

Public housing brought parks, playgrounds, and community centers into slum areas. It gave the transient slum neighborhood stability and continuity. The projects are far better integrated than private housing: in some, Puerto Ricans constitute a third of the population; in others, a half. Public housing is considered such a "good buy" that each year there are 85,000 applications for the 6,000 vacancies (Sexton 1965:37).

The displaced Puerto Ricans who could not obtain a project apartment were forced to spread throughout the metropolitan area, to the East Side and the West Side, uptown and downtown, wherever the descendants of the older immigrants left vacancies in their flight from the city. "Thus because of the housing shortage and slum clearance they rubbed shoulders with everybody in the city" (Glazer and Moynihan 1963:95).

Because entrenched low-income groups were protected by the rent laws, landlords converted their properties into furnished apartments in order to increase their income. The Puerto Ricans had no choice but to accept "subdivided apartments or furnished rooms at exorbitant prices, taking in lodgers to make up the cost" (Handlin 1959:94). The old-law tenements that house Puerto Ricans are frequently neglected by their absentee landlords. Life in these places is an endless, futile struggle against bugs, mice, and rats. Average density is three persons per room, and a four-room apartment may house as many as twelve people. "The conditions . . . are a source of stress in the same sense that they would be for a middle-class suburbanite" (Berle 1958:51).

The neighborhood concentrations that still exist include Puerto Ricans who arrived forty or fifty years ago, and those who were born and brought up in New York. The older migrants generally maintain contact with the island, and provide advice, help and a social model to new migrants. The "ethnic subculture merges migrants into the culture of the city while sheltering them from many of the stresses and strains inherent in migration and in the social system of the city" (Padilla 1958:67). It is cohesive not only because of the common culture but also in self-defense, as a reaction to its rejection by the larger society. Black Puerto Ricans, particularly, rely on the family and group as a source of emotional strength and reinforcement.

However, prejudice in the larger society also "has been a powerful mechanism in splitting the *Hispano* group as a positive and creative source of social and emotional strength." In accepting the values of the mainland, Puerto Ricans accept the devaluation of their own group at the same time as they resent discrimination in employment, housing, and education. Intermediately colored Puerto Ricans who have been reared in New York may remain with the group even when they feel no bond with the island and strongly dislike Puerto Ricans. Race also operates "to separate recent migrants from the older groups of *Hispanos* in the city and from those who are born and reared in New York" (Padilla 1958:56, 80).

Lower-class persons in Puerto Rico are not very much involved in the racial aspects of social mobility, since their mobility is quite limited, but in New York lower-class *Hispano* society is socially mobile (Padilla 1958:75).

The newcomer may rely upon his relatives in New York even more than he did in Puerto Rico, but although he is usually helped by other recent migrants, he is often disappointed by the response from kinsmen who have lived in the city for a number of years. As time passes many Puerto Ricans in New York come to feel responsible only for the nuclear family. New York Puerto Ricans tend to disdain recent migrants with their antiquated ideas about child rearing, the role of women, and obligations to the extended family. In their eagerness to be employed, illiterate, poverty-stricken migrants work for low wages, get into trouble with the law, and increase the prejudice against all Puerto Ricans. Second-generation Puerto Ricans give a "medium" rating to American Negroes including West Indians, and a "high" rating to Americans, Cubans, Italians, Jews, and other European immigrants, but they give a "low" rating to the new Puerto Rican migrant (Sexton 1965:18).

Recent migrants may complain that many of their New York relatives treat them like strangers. The newcomer is often expected to pay for his room and board and to move out as soon as possible. "If one is too poor, one is not really welcome at relatives at all, not even for short visits" (Padilla 1958:60). Nevertheless, most Puerto Ricans do not turn away kinsmen and friends who are jobless and homeless, and visits, both temporary and permanent, are widespread.

Recent migrants are also disliked "by members of all other ethnic groups" (Padilla 1958:83). In the sections of the city where Puerto Ricans, blacks, and Italians live in close proximity, the Italians express open and profound racist feelings.

Race and ethnicity underlie much of the open and hidden conflict in East Harlem, as it always has in the slums of New York's melting pot. The poor, consumed by conflict with the new poor, who are moving in on top of them, often ignore "enemies without" (Sexton 1965:12).

In some areas, such as the lower East Side, "there is strong economic rivalry between the entrenched Italians and the invading Puerto Ricans which creates a far greater social distance between the two groups than mere ethnic differences could" (Mencher 1958:232). In fact, "the Puerto Ricans are closer in life style, religion and attitudes to their Italian rather than their Negro neighbors" (Sexton 1965:10). The children are separated because most of the Italians go to parochial schools, but some intergroup dating and marriage occur.

Great tension exists between recent Puerto Rican migrants and American blacks. The Puerto Ricans regard the blacks as "bad, dangerous and capable of violence against them" (Sexton 1965:18). The blacks disapprove of the migrants because "they accept low-paying jobs and . . . pay landlords large sums to secure apartments" (Padilla 1958:94). However, when blacks and Puerto Ricans live in the same neighborhood for a number of years, they learn "to associate with each other in small groups, become close friends . . . without having their relationships subject to the inter-ethnic tensions of the neighborhood" (Padilla 1958: 94). In the past Puerto Ricans generally refused to participate in civil rights movements because they were unwilling to be identified with blacks. Since the early 1960s, however, the common interests of the two groups have led to some joint political and social action, particularly for the improvement of housing and schools.

The slum neighborhood is a mixture of every ethnic group. Many people are law-abiding, hard-working, conservative, and respectable. But there are also the alcoholics, prostitutes, drug addicts, dope peddlers, sexual perverts, thieves, people who discharge their aggressions destructively, and idle men and boys who teach young children "bad things."

Many slum dwellers live in a generalized state of fear—of being robbed, knifed, attacked, bullied, or having their children injured. The fear colors their whole lives: their ability to learn, to work, to stay sane and healthy, to venture out of their apartments or blocks, to live openly and freely, to be friends with their neighbors, to trust the world, outsiders, themselves (Sexton 1965:116).

Slum residents are very much afraid of the fighting and drug-addict gangs and complain about insufficient police protection. Because of their great fear of the streets, Puerto Rican mothers keep their youngsters in the overcrowded flats summer and winter, and only the disorganized families allow children to play outdoors unsupervised. Children who played freely on the island are nostalgic about their former life. Mothers who are recent migrants escort their children to and from school, for children who speak only Spanish may be attacked by gangs. "The net effect is to force them to learn English and to become 'American'" (Padilla 1958:227).

But the slums also breed many close friendships. Neighbors who live in the same building often cooperate as they try to cope with common problems, and are usually led by men who have lived in the city for many years and speak English well. People join together on a sex and age basis for recreation and sports, but recent migrants are included only in the groups who live in the same building and shop in the same stores. However, the migrants belong to hometown associations, which consist of families from the same town who meet each other for mutual aid and recreation and maintain ties with Puerto Rico, reducing the impact of uprootedness.

The small storekeeper plays as important a role in New York as he does in the San Juan shantytowns and on the coasts. He and his customers are neighbors and friends, and the credit he provides "contributes to making the relationships . . . one of trust, understanding and mutual obligation" (Padilla 1958:14). The lower East Side is an example of communities that are not only the scene of crime and violence, "poor, run-down, alienated, disadvantaged, depressed, underprivileged, garbage strewn," but are also "integrated, dynamic, emergent, hopeful, changing, . . . eager for opportunity" (Grossman 1967:12).

Education

Upward mobility is now achieved mainly through education, and Puerto Ricans are far more concerned about the New York City schools than were the earlier immigrants, for in 1967 "there were high rates of unemployment among Puerto Ricans in the same areas where there were low rates of education" (Fitzpatrick 1969:18). The Puerto Ricans have the lowest level of formal education in the city partially because they come with educational deficits. Despite the tremendous increase in educational facilities in Puerto Rico since 1940, in 1960 more than two-thirds of the rural population had no more than four years of schooling and had the least opportunity on the island to achieve a high school education (Tumin and Feldman 1961:43, 57).

Even the migrant with minimal schooling knows the value of education; a primary goal of migration is the superior educational system in New York. But the migrant's low level of literacy and his inability to implement his aspirations for his children often prevent them from achieving academically. Lower-class Puerto Rican children, in New York, as on the island, have a high rate of school absenteeism. A child may be kept out of school because he does not have the proper clothing, or because of family problems, or because he is needed to act as interpreter for the family. Also, living conditions "combine with the low evaluation given whatever a child does . . . [to] make for interruptions and lack of privacy in studying."

While a child is doing his homework, he will perhaps be asked to run errands, or a parent . . . may speak to him intermittently. . . . In the same room where a child is doing his homework, a television show . . . may be playing, and friends and relatives may have dropped in for a casual chat. . . . Children who sleep in the living room or in the kitchen must wait for visitors to go home and for their parents to retire before they can go to bed (Padilla 1958:209).

The school is the place where the child receives intensive, directed training in becoming American. In addition, when children learn conversational English their status improves in the family. They become interpreters for their parents and their major link to the larger institutions. They also gain status in the neighborhood and the school.

Among school children knowledge of colloquial English and speaking it with the "right accent" are considered a sure way of gaining the recognition and friendship of other children in the neighborhood and the approval of their teachers (Padilla 1958:200).

But the conflicting expectations of the home and the school about a child's behavior create discord in the family. The primary Puerto Rican child-rearing goal is the inculcation of respect, as manifested by the child's docility and complete obedience. The school, however, encourages independence and assertiveness, and when children enact these values at home they are severely punished. Moreover, Puerto Rican migrants prolong child dependency in New York because of their fear of the streets.

If anything Puerto Rican children are kept more dependent on the adults than are their contemporaries in Puerto Rico. In addition to the general cultural emphasis on dependency, the conditions of life in a New York City slum encourage dependency behavior (Mencher 1958:232).

Parents generally expect their children only to complete high school, preferably vocational high school. "Many parents insist that their sons go to a vocational high school in order to learn a trade . . . so that they can get better jobs than their fathers" (Padilla 1958:238), and Puerto Ricans had the greatest percentage increase in the vocational schools from 1962–1963 to 1967–1968. While they "comprised only 22.1 percent of the total school population, they comprised 30.6 percent of those attending vocational high schools . . . but only 13.0 percent of those attending academic schools" in 1967–1968 (Fitzpatrick 1969:7).

In 1967, Puerto Ricans had the lowest enrollment of any group in the City University of New York: 3.3 percent of the matriculated students and 3.9 percent of the nonmatriculated students. Their 1968 enrollment increased by only 0.6 percent over 1967, compared with the black increase of 2.3 percent (Fitzpatrick 1969:10). However, their enrollment at the City University community colleges increased from 7.7 percent in 1969 to 9.6 percent in 1970, when open enrollment was instituted, although at the senior colleges it decreased from 2.5 percent in 1969 to 2.4 percent in 1970. The percentage increase of black enrollment at the City University for this period was 4.5 percent in the community colleges and 2.8 percent in the senior colleges.[4]

In the high schools with the heaviest concentration of Puerto Ricans, the drop-out rate is often as high as 60 percent (Fitzpatrick and Gould 1968:96). Recent adolescent migrants who know little English may be shunned even by other Puerto Ricans, are generally truant, drop out of school as soon as possible, and frequently become delinquent. Students also leave school because they must work in order to help their parents financially. "Whether or not children remain in school seemed to be largely a matter of the individual determination of the parents, regardless of the years of school they themselves had enjoyed" (Berle 1958: 51–52). However, if the prospects for upward mobility were not hampered by discrimination, high-school minority youth would have incentives to "raise the level of their schooling" (Handlin 1959:79).

---

[4]*The New York Times,* March 26, 1971, p. 21.

Puerto Rican children score considerably below national norms in both reading and arithmetic. In the South Bronx, for example, an area with a very high concentration of Puerto Ricans, 52 percent of all sixth-grade pupils were two years below reading level in 1966. The schools they attend are often seriously overcrowded, with double sessions, "excessive use of school facilities . . . and excessive burdens on administrative and teaching staff as well as supporting personnel in health services, remedial programs." Of the 42 schools in the South Bronx with an enrollment of about 60 percent of Puerto Ricans in 1965, "40 were overutilized, some as much as 148 percent" (Fitzpatrick and Gould 1968:95–96).

Most of the elementary schools attended by Puerto Ricans are residentially segregated, although the presence of the many light-skinned Puerto Rican children actually integrates a school. Not only are the teachers often inexperienced, but the teacher and pupil turnover in the slum areas is much greater than in the rest of the city. Parents blame the schools for the poor achievement of the children; the schools blame the parents; the children are inclined to blame themselves.

According to Glazer and Moynihan, "probably no public school system has spent as much money and devoted as much effort to the problems of a group of minority children as the New York public school system has devoted to the Puerto Ricans. There are now hundreds of special personnel to deal with parents, to help teachers, to deal with special problems of students" (Glazer and Moynihan 1963:127). In 1948 the New York City Board of Education recognized the special educational needs of Puerto Rican pupils by establishing the positions of bilingual teacher and non-English coordinator. By 1965 about 270 non-English coordinators were teaching English as a second language to Spanish-speaking pupils and were also training classroom teachers to deal with language problems. In 1967, 142 bilingual teachers in school and community relations were providing resources materials on Puerto Rican culture and fulfilling "for the Puerto Rican parent the image of the schoolteacher which is common in Puerto Rico as the person who is conveniently on hand to settle all problems" (Fitzpatrick 1969:41).

In *The Puerto Rican Study, 1953–1957,* the Board of Education (1958) established the need to find the most effective methods of teaching English to newly arrived Puerto Rican children and to promote "a more rapid and more effective adjustment of Puerto Rican parents and children to the community and of the community to them." To implement their recommendations the Board issued a series of Resource Units and Language Guides for all grades. However, many of the programs that emerged from *The Puerto Rican Study* were largely ineffective because of budget problems, rigid structures and regulations, a lack of adequate personnel, discontinuity, inconsistency, and inadequate evaluation.

From 1948 to 1958 the Board of Education seemed to be guided by a policy of rapid Americanization and not by a desire to preserve the Spanish language of the child. But the problem is how the child can master both English and Spanish. On the island most Puerto Ricans are not really bilingual, although English is taught as a second language, but since Puerto Ricans are American citizens, Spanish is not the language of foreigners. The considerable movement between the island and the mainland "makes it difficult for them to master English if they live periodically on the Island, or to retain their Spanish if they live periodically on the Mainland" (Fitzpatrick 1969:38).

Language is a much more serious problem for the Puerto Ricans than for the earlier immigrants who were not fluent in English, because English is essential for white-collar employment and for dealing effectively with bureaucracies. Also, says Fitzpatrick, "an increasing awareness of the value of bilingualism . . . in any situation has led to a greater concern for helping a child to retain the language of his parents." And again, "Never before has the city been caught in the tension between a determination to teach English and a desire to preserve Spanish" (1969:36, 37).

About 1960 the term "compensatory education" came into use to describe a variety of experimental programs, sponsored by government, private agencies, and foundations, and designed to overcome "assumed deficiencies in the background, functioning, and current experience of children from economically deprived, culturally isolated, and/or ethnically segregated families." But the few evaluations of those programs expressed skepticism about their accomplishments. They represented increased quantitative effort but little improvement of quality since they did not reflect "current thinking relative to learning theory and behavioral organization. . . . when one looks at their impact on academic performance in the target population, it is obvious that compensatory education . . . is either insufficient or irrelevant to the needs of disadvantaged young people" (Gordon and Jablonsky 1968:268).

Also, the various agencies concerned with compensatory education failed to coordinate their data and resources systematically. "As a result, many of the innovations and development . . . remain at the upper level and do not filter down through the rest of the system" (Fantini and Weinstein 1968:181). In addition, it was found that compensatory programs considered only the problems of the poor and did not take into account their strengths, or the differences between their values and those of the middle-class system, especially the values of the teacher (Reissman 1962). In most of the programs and proposals there was a lack of attention to specifically Puerto Rican problems.

As Puerto Ricans suffer the consequences of low educational achievement in their daily lives, they become increasingly frustrated. At its first city-wide conference in April, 1967, the Puerto Rican community expressed great indignation about the inadequate education of its children, and proposed a program that reflected its own educational desires.

[It] demanded bilingual programs, not simply as an instrument for learning English, but as an instrument for developing and preserving the knowledge of Spanish among Puerto Rican children; it demanded the introduction of courses in Puerto Rican culture, literature and history; a much greater involvement of the Puerto Rican community in the planning of school programs for Puerto Rican children; the use of Puerto Rican paraprofessionals as aids to teachers . . . ; and representation on the Board of Education (Fitzpatrick 1969:47).

In January, 1968, Congress passed the Bilingual Education Act providing financial assistance to meet the special educational needs of children with limited English-speaking ability. The Senate hearings on bilingual education programs pinpointed the major problems of the Spanish-speaking child:

A general lack of knowledge on the part of educators regarding teaching two languages together; recognition that Spanish-speaking children are being labeled as slow learners through the device of low IQ scores; and . . . language deprivation as their central handicap (Fitzpatrick 1969:41).

Although representatives of Puerto Rican organizations urged bilingualism as values in themselves, the view that prevailed at the hearings was that Spanish should be taught as an instrument for learning English more easily so that acculturation to American society could be more rapid.

Fitzpatrick believes that the Puerto Ricans can overcome their educational disadvantages by becoming "a political voice . . . pressuring for their rights and interests."

Failure to learn on the part of Puerto Rican children is now analyzed in terms of the organization of the school system and the exercise of power within it. Children are seen as not responsive to the system because the system has not been responsive to the children (1969:58).

A decentralized school system, says Fitzpatrick, would be more flexible and accountable to local communities, and the response of children and of parents would be more favorable and productive.

Although the Puerto Rican community favors decentralization, it is concerned about its own representation at the community level. Puerto

Ricans must share community boards with other minority groups, particularly blacks, because of their "social, political and geographical proximity," but this association "has not always been congenial" (Fitzpatrick 1969:63), especially over the question of leadership. In March, 1968, the Puerto Rican Leadership Conference opposed the complete control of education by local boards "because certain extremist groups push out minority groups like Puerto Ricans and other whites."[5]

But despite their many problems, Fitzpatrick points out, "there are evidences of considerable improvement educationally and occupationally among second generation Puerto Ricans" (1969:3).

Religion

In both race and religion, Puerto Ricans are a swing group, part Negro and part white, part Catholic and part Protestant (Sexton 1965:77).

Although churches abound in the slum areas and more adults are involved with a church than with any other voluntary association, the evangelist, Billy Graham, found that in 1960 more than half a million Spanish-speaking people in New York were "unchurched" (Glazer and Moynihan 1963:107).

The vast majority of Puerto Ricans on the island and the mainland are Catholics, but they become involved in other religions because they are looking for a community that meets their needs, not because they have doctrinal differences with Catholicism. Indeed, many Puerto Ricans "are convinced that Catholicism has made their culture a gentle and compassionate one, and the people serene and unobsessed by material pursuits" (Sexton 1965:77). Their weak affiliation with Catholicism on the island is partially due to the almost complete absence of the Church from many of the rural villages.

Unlike the Catholic immigrants from Europe, Puerto Ricans have no national parish of their own, partly because they are dispersed throughout New York. Also, "there is a widespread conviction that a much more positive effort toward integration within the territorial parish will hasten the adjustment of the Puerto Rican to the customs of the mainland parish" (Fitzpatrick 1955:415). However, in the mixed parishes the Church treads an uneasy course between the interests of the Italians and the Puerto Ricans.

The proportion of Spanish-speaking priests to the Catholic Puerto

---

[5]*The New York Times,* March 26, 1968.

Rican population is less than a third of what it is for other New York Catholics, and the migrants cannot find a community in parishes where the priests do not speak Spanish. Moreover, few of the Spanish-speaking priests are Puerto Rican, whereas in the more than 270 Protestant churches with Spanish services the ministers are almost all Puerto Rican, and they have closer relations with their congregations than the Catholic priests have with their parishioners (Senior 1961:108–109). The capacities of the Church are weak in the very areas in which the migrants have great needs, that is, "in creating a surrounding supporting community to replace the extended families broken by city life, and to supply a social setting for those who feel lost and lonely in the great city" (Glazer and Moynihan 1963:104).

Only about 16 percent of Puerto Rican children attend parochial schools, "a much smaller percentage than for any other Catholic group in the city" (Glazer and Moynihan 1963:107). On the lower East Side, for example, the parochial school is overwhelmingly Italian "and there is considerable opposition to taking in Puerto Ricans" (Mencher 1958: 277). But the Church assists the migrants through its settlement houses, Catholic Charities, and other church-related organizations. A third to a half of the clients of Catholic Charities' family and child-service agencies are Puerto Rican (Glazer and Moynihan 1963:107).

About 20 percent of the Puerto Rican population in New York are Protestant, but 50 percent of the Protestant Puerto Ricans are regular churchgoers, compared with 25 percent of the Catholics (Senior 1961: 108). About 10,000 Puerto Rican Protestants have their own all-Spanish churches, staffed by Puerto Rican ministers. "Evangelical zeal puts most Anglo-Saxon Protestantism to shame, and the willingness to spend money to support the church is also great" (Glazer and Moynihan 1963:105).

Some members of the white Protestant clergy with democratic-socialist beliefs run community-wide programs in the slums. The ministers often live in the areas they serve, and they stress grass-roots organization and community decision-making in housing and education. Many neighborhood churches have supplanted the political leader in establishing more direct channels of communication between the community and government agencies, in their support of political issues, and in social welfare work, especially with recent migrants.

The Pentecostal and other revivalist sects arouse the greatest fervor among low-income Puerto Ricans. According to Glazer and Moynihan, in 1960 there were 240 self-supporting evangelical churches, with a membership of at least 25,000, which conducted daily services. Many have grown quite large from their tiny storefront beginnings, and have full-time ministers, almost all Puerto Rican, who have risen from the membership. The Pentecostal churches "derive their strength from Catholicism's weakness . . . the tight congregation is one of the most important expressions of a community that is found among Puerto Ricans in New York" (Glazer and Moynihan 1963:105–106). The revivalist sects specialize "in togetherness, friendliness, activity, excitation, warmth—special low-income Puerto Rican and Negro qualities" (Sexton 1965:73). They perform for the Puerto Ricans the functions that the Black Muslims perform for the blacks, but do not organize by means of protest and race conflict.

The membership in these churches, however, is often transient. The father, who is much more dominant in the revivalist sects than in the Catholic or traditional Protestant churches, may lead his family into a sect one day and as quickly lead it out again. Many of the Puerto Rican nuclear families, which tend to be disorganized, are members of the sects. The better organized extended families are generally Catholic, and "are less likely to need the help that the Protestant churches offer" (Mencher 1958:77).

Puerto Rican parents who have no church affiliations often send their children to a church of their own choice "as a means of furthering their adjustment to the expectations of the wider society" (Handlin 1959:108). Members of the same family sometimes attend churches of different faiths, and parents tend to resent attempts to bring them into the church their children attend. The second generation, however, seems to be turning to the traditional faith as part of the process of becoming Americanized.

Regardless of their religious affiliations or lack of them, most Puerto Ricans believe in the power of the saints and the Virgin, and an unrecorded number practice Spiritualism, as in Puerto Rico. Like other working-class people, they generally believe that destiny and chance determine the course of an individual's life, and they employ various magical techniques to change chronic bad luck.

Health

Incentives to migration include not only prospects for occupational and educational advancement, but also the superior health and medical facilities of New York. Illness creates overwhelming problems in all aspects of the migrant's daily life. He views good health as "a gift from God," the prerequisite for the good life, and regards illness "as a punishment for wrong doing, a work of evil, or a trick of fate" (Padilla 1958:275).

The illness of a parent creates especially serious problems. When the male breadwinner in a nuclear family falls ill and income is reduced, "the mother's potential role as chief breadwinner . . . is considered more threatening to family integrity and masculine self-respect than acceptance of public assistance" (Berle 1958:57). The wife's illness disrupts the nuclear family perhaps even more than the husband's, for the man believes he is incapable of doing "woman's work." However, migrants in New York have been forced to modify their view of male and female roles when confronted with crises. "One may hear young recent migrant fathers and mothers say that in this country it is important for a man to learn how to change a baby or how to take care of a home in case the wife falls ill" (Padilla 1958:299).

Illness "is a powerful mechanism . . . in reestablishing and solidifying social bonds that have been strained or disrupted," for the sick person is forgiven all his faults and errors. Illness is the "basis for human sympathy and cooperation, and is an effective means of getting people together and stimulating their charity" (Padilla 1958:277). People in different ethnic groups who are normally hostile to one another go out of their way to help or visit a sick child or an older person.

Puerto Ricans generally believe that health is better in New York than in Puerto Rico, but the change from a rural area on the island to a different climate and culture in a large city creates great susceptibility to many types of illness. The incidence of hospitalization during the first year following migration is very high, both for street accidents and for major respiratory disease, pertussis, and tuberculosis. Puerto Rican migrants have a higher incidence of tuberculosis than any other ethnic group in New York, and their fear of this disease is so great that its existence is often denied. Sometimes a family never recovers from the setback resulting from an initial accident or illness.

The rate of growth of Puerto Rican children in the early years is about the same as that of other Americans, but after the age of ten "they do not appear to keep pace with the previous development." Puerto Rican children born in New York have a high rate of hospital admissions, especially for major respiratory infections, which appear to be most numerous in dwellings that are not centrally heated and where three or four persons sleep in one room (Berle 1958:38, 96).

Older migrants, who are most preoccupied with illness, place considerable stock in folk medicine. Many believe that illness is caused by the witchcraft of envious people, for "envy is considered a powerful destructive force" (Padilla 1958:283). Although young adults, whether reared in Puerto Rico or New York, rely primarily on scientific medicine and do not attribute the illnesses of their own babies to *mal de ojo,* they carefully avoid "casting the evil eye" on their relatives and friends, and refrain from complimenting a mother on her baby's physical appearance or health.

Illness calls for action and attack. Home remedies, such as purgatives, are tried first. But if they are not efficacious and an illness is acute, or the waiting period for a clinic appointment is too long, the individual may visit the emergency ward of a hospital. Injections inspire optimism, for they are believed to cure most illnesses. If scientific medical treatment fails, however, the spirits may be blamed, and the next recourse is the *espiritista*. Even Puerto Ricans who are reared in New York occasionally consult a Spiritualist medium (Mencher 1958:143–144), as do other native New Yorkers.

Despite the concern about health, Puerto Ricans often ignore preventive health care. When the health department publicized its cancer detection program, only those Puerto Ricans responded "who had an overwhelming anxiety about their health" (Mencher 1958:175). The modest Puerto Rican woman is very reluctant to undergo a breast or pelvic examination, even by a female doctor, and the Puerto Rican man, who associates nudity with sexuality, often refuses to be examined by a female doctor.

Puerto Ricans may go to a clinic for a series of visits when they are concerned about nonhealth problems, but they fail to use preventive facilities mainly because of "a general lack of future orientation that characterizes blue-collar workers." Since illness is related to work dysfunction, only symptoms that are incapacitating create concern. However, working men and housewives with small children cannot spend long hours waiting for appointments in the different departments of a clinic. And even when illness is serious, they will "hesitate to utilize agencies or facilities which they perceive as unsympathetic" (Rosenblatt and Suchman 1964:344–345). "Medical personnel and Puerto Rican families were observed to operate at times from entirely different premises, and this lack of reciprocal understanding was a source of frustration to both groups" (Berle 1958:115). But Puerto Ricans were "responsive and cooperative where medical personnel expressed personal interest in them and provided continuity of treatment" (Berle 1958:195).

For the period 1948 to 1951 the crude rate of mental illness of Puerto Ricans in New York, 157.7 per 100,000, was somewhat higher than for the total metropolitan population, which was 144.5. However, the rate of first admissions of Puerto Ricans with schizophrenia to hospitals was very high compared with the total population. For Puerto Rican males it was 114.3, twice that of the total male population, and for Puerto Rican females it was 85.6, compared with 54.5 for the total female population. Malzberg noted that "the rate of first admissions with dementia praecox [schizophrenia], when corrected for age and sex proportions, was 99.4 per 100,000 for Puerto Ricans, and 55.6 for the non-Puerto Ricans." He attributed the significantly higher incidence of schizophrenia among Puerto Ricans to their language handicap, their severely limited occupational opportunities, and their segregation in areas that were substandard in housing and health (1956:269).

The 1967 mental illness admissions data showed that while schizophrenia had increased only slightly for Puerto Rican women, it had increased to 121.8 for men, along with a great increase of psychoses and psychoneuroses (Fitzpatrick and Gould 1968:59). Many schizophrenic Puerto Ricans manifest a syndrome typical of anxious and frustrated individuals. The unskilled, uneducated migrant may be unable to reconcile his aspirations with his limited employment opportunities. Mental illness releases him from the obligation to continue to strive for an impossible goal, and justifies his failure and desire for care without loss of self-respect. But the mainland practice of treating disturbed people outside of the context of family and neighborhood probably aggravates the condition of schizophrenic Puerto Ricans, especially since Puerto Rican families have a great capacity to cope with mental illness.

In addition, mainland physicians who are unfamiliar with Puerto Rican culture occasionally diagnose as a symptom of serious personality disorder the "Puerto Rican syndrome," the *ataque*. This is widespread among low-income Puerto Ricans both on the island and the mainland, and represents "a popular and conventional reaction to overwhelming catastrophe" (Berle 1958:160). It is expressed by sudden, violent, uncommunicative hyperkinesis in situations which an individual cannot handle—the hospitalization of a child, a death, or a funeral. The *ataque* has also been associated with the "hysterical" behavior which "seems to be more common and much more generally accepted in Puerto Rico than in the United States" (Rothenberg 1964:962). It may be a method of expressing aggression and hostility, which are strongly repressed and suppressed in the culture.

Puerto Ricans comprised 33 percent of the enrollment in the "Special Schools" for children with behavior problems in 1967, although they accounted for only 22.1 percent of the total New York City school enrollment (Fitzpatrick and Gould 1968:16). But very few of the psychiatrists at the Bureau of Child Guidance of the Board of Education speak Spanish. And only two mental health centers in the metropolitan area are completely staffed by Spanish-speaking personnel. Spokesmen for the Puerto Rican community complain bitterly about the lack of Spanish-speaking staff and the absence of programs to train such staff in the great majority of the hospitals serving Spanish-speaking neighborhoods. They insist that "the lack of language is a symbol in many cases of lack of sensitivity to the culture and way of life of the Spanish-speaking people," and results in "the evident overemphasis on physical treatment and confinement in the case of the poor" (Fitzpatrick and Gould 1968:25).

The treatment of mental illness is a social-class as well as an ethnic problem, for upper-class professionals appear to be seriously biased in their treatment of lower-class people. The professional view of mental health, as revealed in the literature, showed the influence of the Protestant ethic thirty years ago (Davis 1938:55–56). A more recent analysis of the literature showed that the mental health movement was still "unwittingly propagating a middle-class ethic under the guise of science," and that this view, which "represents the functional equivalent of religion," is now even more influential than it was earlier because it is being disseminated by the greatly expanded mass media (Gursslin, Hunt and Roach 1964:63, 64). However, since it is acknowledged that socially structured strains constitute a primary source of mental disorder, the mental health movement may be supporting a social system that is producing a high incidence of mental illness. Also, the lower-class individual who accepts the middle-class model of the mentally healthy person, which differs markedly from the lower-class prototype, may become seriously disorganized. Thus the mental health movement may be producing the very effects it is intended to combat (Gursslin, Hunt and Roach 1964:64).

Those who treat the mental illness of the poor have great power, but the poor who are treated lack power.

Those in control of the mental health facilities determine the definitions, the methods and condition of treatment. They can confine those who are weak or segregate them for treatment. They can apply the system favorably to cases they understand, or unfavorably to those they do not understand. What is crucial for the poor is the fact that they have no access to strategic control (Fitzpatrick and Gould 1968:82).

During the past few years the professional community has become increasingly self-critical. At the 1968 convention of the American Orthopsychiatric Association, Dr. Thomas H. Linton said, "There are few professionals in the mental health field who are unaware of the chaos, disorganization and professional exploitation which deeply and tragically scar our work in this field" (Fitzpatrick and Gould 1968:82).

Recently the New York City Community Mental Health Board began to build comprehensive community mental health centers, and one center is already operating in Maimonides Hospital in a section of Brooklyn with a large Puerto Rican population. Since Puerto Ricans tend to regard mental health centers as insane asylums where the *loco* are incarcerated for life, doctors and other staff members visit families to explain the nature of their services and become involved in community activities and antipoverty programs. Neighborhood people, trained as aides, link the center to the community. The center staff and some of the teachers in the area also work on the low reading level of Spanish-speaking children, which aggravates tensions and frustrations in school.

Lincoln Hospital, in the most densely populated Puerto Rican section of the Bronx, cooperated with the Albert Einstein College of Medicine in pioneering the integration of mental health services with those related to housing, welfare, religion, etc., for it views mental illness in relation to poverty, migration and the tensions of rapidly changing neighborhoods. Lincoln Hospital has identified the strengths of the Puerto Rican community in their hometown associations, the Pentecostal churches and Spiritualism.

The Hospital has discovered unexpected strengths in the Puerto Rican community for the management of people with mental disorders; has inaugurated an anthropological study of spiritualists and the practice of spiritualism because these often play an effective role in assisting people with mental health difficulties (Fitzpatrick and Gould 1968:107).

The Gouverneur Hospital on the lower East Side, another area with a large Puerto Rican population, relates mental health problems to the total social and cultural context of the individual's life, and according to Fitzpatrick and Gould, "is remarkably suited to be helpful to new and strange residents from Puerto Rico and elsewhere." It operates on the theory that "what is called mental retardation or mental illness may be a lack of cognitive development, namely the presence of conceptual and information gaps in people who because of such deficits are unable to cope with the complexities of today's urban world." When a patient receives help from a number of agencies, the caseworkers from all the agencies form a committee and meet, preferably in the patient's home, to determine the central issue. When Spanish-speaking patients are involved, the team usually includes Spanish-speaking professionals, and "there is little danger that a Puerto Rican will be committed to a mental hospital for something which may be a cultural practice, or a serious interfamilial problem, or a cognitive deficiency" (1968:112–115).

Marriage and the Family

Although industrialization and urbanization are gradually changing traditional values and roles in Puerto Rico, they change much more rapidly in New York. The institutions of marriage and the family, however, are particularly resistant to change. In fact, the Puerto Rican migrant in New York may cling even more tenaciously to the traditional lifeways as a buffer against the sharp conflicts that confront him between the extended and the nuclear family, the large family and the small, the consensual union and legal marriage, authoritarian and egalitarian conjugal roles.

Given the weakness of the Puerto Rican sense of identity and of the ethnic community, the extended family is a most important source of support for the recent migrant. This is particularly the case for the migrant from the sugar-growing coasts, where the extended family is very strong, and it is "predominantly from the sugar-producing parts of the island" (Mencher 1958:32–33), that the recent migration has come. The migrants continue the coastal matrifocal pattern in New York, where women rely, even more than in Puerto Rico, on female relatives for a mutual exchange of services. Without the help of her relatives the migrant wife finds it very difficult to cope with the children and the household. "According to the norms of the . . . subculture from which the migrants come," the nuclear family is "a form of social disorganization" (Mencher 1958:2).

The bonds among members of the extended family are fortified by ritual kinship, which provides every child with godparents who are usually relatives either in New York or on the island. In an emergency an aunt may be more willing to take care of an orphaned niece or nephew who is also a godchild.

With migration to New York the practice of having children live with their close-kin godparents in Puerto Rico, or of sending them to stay with their kin-godparents in New York, has become quite common . . . particularly . . . among husbandless mothers . . . in search of employment (Padilla 1958:122).

In New York the housing shortage operates to separate members of the extended family and public housing management ignores family relationships in tenant selection. In addition, Puerto Ricans who have grown up in New York may feel no obligations to recent migrants who are poor, although they generally sustain relationships with kin they have known since childhood, and with relatives in Puerto Rico who are rich or socially important. While the extended family is still the ideal, in practice it is warded off, and the newcomers "find the rules for family living are changing right before their eyes, and new rules . . . develop regardless of whether they approve . . . or live by them" (Padilla 1958:147).

A Columbia University anthropological study of 375 Puerto Rican families on the lower East Side found that about half the families were extended and lived in the same apartment, in different apartments in the same building, or in nearby buildings or streets (Mencher 1958:84). If the migrants cannot find quarters close to the extended family, or if they lack family connections in New York, they try to move close to hometown friends. But if they have neither relatives nor friends, "the majority of Puerto Rican residents are quite isolated from their neighbors, including other Puerto Ricans" (Mencher 1958:23–24). Since interracial marriage is common among the coastal sugarcane workers, the racially mixed migrants in the nuclear family remain marginal in the slum communities of New York. Lacking community integration, they suffer "a chronic status frustration [which] leads into social anomie and family disruption" (Seda-Bonilla 1966:163).

The Midtown Manhattan Study found an inverse relationship between the degree of previous attachment to the homeland and ease of acculturation among immigrants in New York. Its Puerto Rican sample, geographically isolated from the main settlements in the city, was far more attached to the homeland and had twice the rate of mental impairment of European immigrants with the same family income (Srole et al. 1962:292–293).

According to Glazer and Moynihan, the lower-class Puerto Rican family is not a source of great strength even under the best of circumstances. Both the Puerto Rican and the European peasant family are patriarchal and authoritarian, but the Polish and Italian family are more stable. In Puerto Rico "concubinage and sexual adventurism on the part of the men . . . meant that children often grew up in confused family settings, . . . which introduced a strain between husbands and wives" (1963:88–89).

In the Columbia study sample, fewer than a third of the marriages were consensual, although half the informants reported two or more marriages (Mencher 1958:100). In most cases the father continues to support his children even when he is living with another woman who is bearing him a second family. When a woman remarries, she is more likely to keep the children from the first marriage if she has an extended family on which to rely, but if the family is nuclear she may send the children to a relative in Puerto Rico.

The consensual union is accepted in the slums of New York, and the children of such unions are not stigmatized. But the larger society penalizes the consensual union; for example, those who are not legally married are excluded from the housing projects. Middle-class Puerto Ricans especially condemn the nonlegal union because they believe it increases prejudice against all Puerto Ricans. "Hence in the context of the slum the Puerto Rican consensual marriage is protected from some of the stresses placed upon it by the larger society" (Padilla 1958:103).

However, if the marital status of Puerto Ricans who return to the island is typical of those who remain on the mainland, than a concomitant of acculturation is a decline in consensual unions. According to the 1960 census, return migrant women living in consensual unions comprised only 5.1 percent and return migrant males, only 6 percent of the total ever married, compared with 11.2 percent of ever-married women and 12.6 percent of ever-married men at least fourteen years old living in common-law marriages in Puerto Rico. Consensual unions among Puerto Ricans on the mainland appear to have declined and legal marriages increased because civil and religious facilities for marriage are more available in the United States than in certain areas of Puerto Rico, and because the United States is less tolerant of consensual unions (Hernández-Alvarez 1967:84–85).

At the same time, the number of illegitimate births among Puerto Rican women, as well as among black and white women, has increased greatly. A recent labor union survey reported an increase of 112.5 percent in illegitimate births in New York City for the period between 1957 and 1967. Among Puerto Ricans such births rose from 10.7 to 21.9 percent, compared with a rise from 1.7 to 5.3 percent among whites, and from 24 to 38.3 percent among blacks. For all ethnic groups there appeared to be "growing rejection of the idea that a stable, legal family is the fundamental socializing agency in our society" (Kihss 1968a:21).

Recent migrants seem to indulge in "sexual misconduct" more freely in New York than in Puerto Rico. Women become "loose and lost" (Padilla 1958:105) and have affairs with married men. But while Puerto Ricans tolerate male adultery, they strongly disapprove of female adultery. Women who have children from casual liaisons with a succession of men are universally condemned, even by their families, and their children are stigmatized as illegitimate.

According to the Bureau of Labor Statistics, "The Puerto Rican family living in New York City tends to be significantly larger in size than families among the white non-Puerto Ricans" (1968:5). Most "adjusted" Puerto Rican families, that are not on relief and are intact, are small. "The bigger family may not get into a good apartment or a housing project. The crowding in a small apartment may mean more illness and poor management of children" (Glazer and Moynihan 1963:117–118).

Most Puerto Ricans are not influenced by the attitudes of the Catholic Church toward birth control and want no more than three children. Other factors, however, interfere with the use of contraception. Men associate male contraceptives with prostitutes and refuse to use them with their wives. Women put off getting free supplies because of the long waiting periods in the clinics. Strong concern over family size typically occurs late because of lack of experience with long-range planning. But the greatest obstacle to family planning, both on the island and the mainland, is the communication barrier between low-income husbands and wives, particularly on matters of sex. Thus, abortions are performed secretly by midwives. But sterilization, the method most opposed by the Catholic Church, is considered the safest, the most natural and direct means of contraception, and many migrants return to Puerto Rico for *la operación.*

In a study of seventy-five native Puerto Rican women with children, Berle (1958:138) found that twenty were sterilized. A recent study conducted in prenatal, gynecological, and family-planning clinics on the lower East Side found that out of 100 Puerto Rican women randomly sampled, "42 wanted sterilization, a strikingly high percentage." Although 68 percent of the husbands "rejected the idea of sterilization, . . . this did not deter the wives" (Handler 1968:25). Puerto Ricans reared in New York reject sterilization, associating it with recent migrants (Padilla 1958:111–112).

The Latin American family engenders different kinds of stress for the male and for the female. Male problems center around submission to and resentment against authority, anxiety about achieving *machismo,* and difficulty in overcoming dependence on women. Female problems arise from the restrictions on girls to ensure a proper marriage, and from the role conflicts arising out of sociocultural change (Díaz-Guerrero 1955:411–417). Both male and female problems are exacerbated in New York by the unfavorable socioeconomic status of the male migrant, the woman's improved economic position, and by American conjugal role models.

In his relationship with his wife, the traditional Puerto Rican wavers between the role of husband and the role of son.

He is dependent and demanding; he leaves most practical matters at home to be handled by his wife; he feels that his duty ends with being the provider. At the same time he feels displaced by his children and has difficulty in finding a way to become integrated into the family (Minuchin et al. 1967:239).

When the man is able to support his family adequately his authority is unchallenged. But when supplementary income is provided by his wife, a child, or the welfare department, his authority decreases, and when he is totally unable to earn money, he has little or no authority in the home. He may then try to validate his masculinity by sexual conquests and "adolescent-type activities directed against his wife (and women in general)" (Minuchin et al. 1967:239), such as excessive drinking and gambling. This is also the male role model in the culture of poverty in New York. Brown predicted that social delinquency, mental illness, and alcoholism would increase rapidly among Puerto Rican men in New York "unless their needs for social recognition and participation, for group recreation, for regular and better-paid employment, and for more satisfying family roles can be met" (1961:188).

The wife feels that her husband constantly exploits her, and that she has no alternative but to leave him.

She seems to deny her real strength, actually manifested quite clearly in her practical adaptation to the new culture, her management of the new household, her relationships to her children, and her ability to press for role revision on the part of her man (Minuchin et al. 1967:240).

The traditional Puerto Rican wife often works from morning to night, unless she has a relative to help her. Family members usually have their meals at different times, and the mother may cook rice and beans for the father and "American" food for the children. The father eats by himself so that he will not be disturbed, and the mother eats alone after she has served everyone in the household. Regardless of the condition of the building, the good housewife must keep the apartment spotlessly clean. Her husband rarely compliments her on its appearance; the absence of criticism is praise enough.

The man's wages "are already consumed or owed by the time he gets paid" (Padilla 1958:153), and the housewife may exaggerate the needs of the family and the amount of the debts in order to get some money for herself. Marketing is one of the very few activities permitting social contact with other women in the neighborhood, for the traditional woman stays home most of the time. The husband is a free agent and comes and goes as he pleases.

But migrants who were married in Puerto Rico find that their wives change in New York. Since employment is easier to find, many more Puerto Rican women work in New York, and since welfare assistance is much larger than in Puerto Rico, they become much more independent. Also, the female role model is less subordinate in New York. When the Puerto Rican man says he has less authority over his wife in New York because he can be taken to the police or to court more easily than in Puerto Rico, he is rationalizing his inability to cope with his wife's greater independence.

Puerto Rican women brought up in New York are not viewed as potentially good wives because they also insist on role desegregation. They want their husbands to help with household chores and the care of children, and they believe that husband and wife should share family problems and recreation. But the men reared in New York often subscribe to the traditional values about women's role and thus they prefer to marry recent migrants. Female migrants, in turn, regard Puerto Rican men who have grown up in New York as potentially good husbands because they do help their wives and do not "run around" with other women, and, unlike the recent male migrant, they are not threatened when their wives work outside the home and contribute financially to the household.

In Puerto Rico, "the old myths of the family, with their blueprint for family organization, coexist with emergent forms being created by socio-economic change" (Minuchin et al. 1967:240). But in the New York slum subculture, the Puerto Rican family experiences the clash between the traditional and the new much more forcefully. However, even the disorganized families "still seem to have some access, however tenuous, to a stabilizing cultural tradition" (Minuchin et al. 1967:237). Compared with disorganized black families, male and female roles are more stable. Women compromise "with their desires for greater personal freedom in order to support their husbands' needs for family dominance and self-respect" (Brown 1961:260). And when the husband leaves, his absence is keenly felt; "the mother's relatedness to and incompleteness without the adult male seems to come across to the Puerto Rican child much more clearly than it does to the Negro child" (Minuchin et al. 1967:236).

Important sources of support and assistance for Puerto Rican migrants in large American cities are the evangelical churches and the Spiritualist mediums "because they are ties with the old ways and can be employed to maintain family intactness" (Minuchin et al. 1967:241).

Child Rearing and the Second Generation

Changes in child-rearing practices are related to both the structure and the status of the family. Puerto Rican migrants in the extended family appear to accept change in child rearing more readily than those in the nuclear family, who cling to traditional patterns as their only anchor in the new society. The nuclear families that most resist change are those with the least status: the families without a male head, those in which the children are the result of casual liaisons, those that have dark-skinned members, and those that depend completely on welfare assistance. Half the families in the Columbia study "manifest a need to rise socially" (Mencher 1958:167), and the families with a strong drive for upward mobility, more often the extended families, insist least on traditional behavior. But even in the upwardly mobile, integrated, extended family, migrants face many child-rearing problems.

In the more remote rural areas of Puerto Rico the mother may still be delivered by a midwife, but in New York she starts to visit a prenatal clinic during the third or fourth month of pregnancy, generally gives birth in a municipal hospital, and takes her babies to a pediatric clinic for checkups and immunizations.

If the mother already has two or three children, she is unhappy about another pregnancy, which will further restrict her activities, and she vents her resentment freely upon her husband and children. In the extended family, the children turn to "significant others," particularly the grandmother. With little opportunity for employment, either in Puerto Rico or New York, the grandmother has a minimum of authority, and is a source of comfort to the grandchildren.

Despite her previous dissatisfaction, the mother usually accepts the new baby warmly and resumes normal relations with her husband and children. In New York exclusive bottle-feeding is almost universal among low-income Puerto Ricans, permitting the use of a mother-surrogate and greater freedom for the mother. Bottle-feeding may continue until the child starts school and even after. When there are several preschool children, each has his own bottle. Pacifiers are also used extensively, and oral dependency lasts for a much longer period than is usual on the mainland. Eating and sleeping are largely unscheduled, and children are not trained for the time-oriented larger society.

The modesty training of the little girl starts very early and continues through adolescence. But in New York the baby girl is sometimes left uncovered, and the father or an uncle may change her diaper, which rarely occurs among the lower classes in Puerto Rico. The practice of fondling and joking about the male genitals is declining; many mothers keep the little boy covered in accordance with "American standards of decency" (Mencher 1958:130–131). Where early male modesty is not observed, the nudity of little boys is associated with the transmission of gastrointestinal infection from the fecal contamination of floors, hands, and toys (Brown 1961:259).

When the child begins to walk or when a new baby is born, infancy ends and childhood starts, usually abruptly and harshly, with toilet training. In the coffee highlands and the sugar-growing coasts, toilet training is gradual and permissive, but in New York the mother demands sharply different behavior from the young child than from the baby, and physical punishment plays a large part in toilet training. A year-old child may be beaten for a toilet lapse, or ridiculed by elder siblings. The severity of punishment is at least partially due to the frustrations created by crowded quarters, for in the project apartments toilet training appears to be more permissive. Enuresis sometimes lasts until the age of ten and causes considerable friction between parents and children, although no attempt is made to stop the bedtime bottle. In the tenements the lack of a private toilet, the locked hall toilets with their high seats, the cold, and the fear of rats probably underlie the persistence of bed-wetting.

In a small apartment the two youngest children may have to sleep in the parents' bedroom and, as in the rural areas, children become sexually aware at an early age. Yet adults insist that children never ask questions about sex, and parents seldom volunteer sexual information.

The traditional Puerto Rican mother is warm, but restrictive and authoritarian. She keeps the child bound to her by deliberately fostering dependency, especially in New York, where 85 percent of Puerto Rican children are kept in the house most of the time. "Only after years in New York do parents accept the idea that young children can play outdoors without becoming a problem" (Padilla 1958:195). Since mothers and children are in the house so much of the time, television plays a very important part in their acculturation. The mother's discipline is neither very consistent nor effective, but when the father enforces obedience at her request, she allies herself with the children against him. The father demands deference and instant obedience. But while he is traditionally more distant with his sons, in New York "an equalizing agent is at work on the affectional relationships between parents and children" (Mencher 1958:184).

Parents rarely consult children even on matters that directly affect them. Without considering their desires, parents buy very expensive toys as holiday gifts and display them prominently, for they "function as items of conspicuous consumption" (Padilla 1958:211). But the children are allowed to play with them only on special occasions. Children are punished when they break a costly toy, but parents sometimes destroy children's playthings when they are disobedient. Children rarely own anything of their own. The rural pattern of sharing is continued in New York, and children who do not share with siblings, cousins, and visitors are considered badly brought up. Traditional parents regard play as a nuisance to be outgrown as soon as possible, and seldom participate in games with children for fear of losing their respect. However, the more acculturated parents buy picture and storybooks for preschool children and young parents now take a more active interest in children's games.

Some of the major stresses of the Puerto Rican children derive from the dysfunction of traditional child-rearing practices in New York. As in Puerto Rico, the young child is considered to be *sin capacidad,* a passive creature who is molded entirely by parental training. Individual achievement is encouraged only as a means of helping the family, and maturity is not related to initiative. *"Capacidad* is achieved through an ever-increasing respect for parents and the growth of ability to handle life situations in approved ways" (Padilla 1958:185).

Respeto, the cornerstone of Puerto Rican child rearing, "is tangled with demands for sheer obedience, so that it is used to sabotage a child's autonomy." In the name of respect, the Puerto Rican value of *cariño,* "a great capacity for tenderness, is subordinated to an undue emphasis on producing a docile child . . . and under the aegis of respect for the parents, the child is subjected to great disrespect" (Minuchin et al. 1967:238–239).

While aggression is constructively channeled in some of the rural subcultures, it is harshly curbed in New York because parents believe it creates a bad impression. Neither offensive nor defensive aggression is permitted, and when siblings fight with each other, both are punished. No matter what kind of punishment parents inflict, counteraggression by children is not tolerated. But aggression is a component of successful upward mobility in an industrialized society, and its total suppression is maladaptive, especially in the slum subculture, where children must be aggressive to survive on the streets. Children are confused by the conflicting standards of behavior in the home and in the community, and they dichotomize their responses. "There is 'good' behavior at home, involving a submissive attitude with repression of resentment; and expressions of aggression and anti-social acting-out in the school and on the street" (Minuchin et al. 1967:240).

Punishment is meted out capriciously and is proportionate to the degree of anger and embarrassment which the child causes the parent. The reasons for punishment are seldom given, but good behavior is taken for granted and is not rewarded. Beating, scolding, ridicule, and criticism are the usual means of punishment, but deprivation, ostracism, and withdrawal of love are rarely used. Children are permitted to withdraw psychologically when they are punished; the crowded quarters prevent physical withdrawal. Women who work outside the home and share child rearing with the father and relatives use physical punishment less and verbal guidance more than women who stay at home, even those in extended families. Punishment is most severe in families with the least mobility and status.

The migrants say that their greatest difficulties in New York center around the children, especially the daughters. "In Puerto Rico, despite rapid urbanization and industrialization, . . . it is perfectly clear how one raises children." The girls are carefully watched, warned to guard their virginity so that they will be able to enter into a legal marriage, "and relatively early escape from this restrictive stifling atmosphere into marriage and motherhood" (Glazer and Moynihan 1963:123). In New York the girl is also expected to become a *señorita* at adolescence, but whereas in San Juan the children of the rural migrants seldom complete more than six years of schooling, in New York adolescents of both sexes are attending high school and preparing for jobs, and the sex roles are more blurred than in Puerto Rico.

Also, in the New York slums there is no one model for adolescent behavior. "There are Negro, Jewish and Italian models, . . . as well as the American models of the welfare workers and the settlement houses." The social worker or minister arranges dances and other co-educational activities and tries to introduce young people to "proper American behavior" by "teaching them how to relate to each other in ways that are not purely sexual and exploitative." To the Puerto Rican parents these activities seem to be "simply shocking invitations to premature pregnancy," but daughters who are prevented from attending them become resentful at treatment to which their classmates and friends are not subjected. "Very often the children who go to the centers and the church activities are the ones from the most disorganized families, where the effort to raise them in proper fashion has been given up, and they are allowed to run wild" (Glazer and Moynihan 1963:123–124).

The training of Puerto Rican boys is marked by very sharp discontinuities. After a more indulged infancy, when they are encouraged to be more aggressive than girls, boys must then become just as obedient, for they are not permitted to imitate the dominant, aggressive *macho* until adolescence. Although fathers use the belt indiscriminately on sons and daughters, mothers scold girls before they resort to beating them, but do not hesitate to beat sons without warning, since they believe boys are naturally more aggressive and must be treated more roughly. The more acculturated families no longer sharply characterize boys as aggressive and girls as passive. The idea that children are all the same comes out in the data collected by the Columbia study (Mencher 1958:204–205).

In Puerto Rico boys are "taught to be proper males . . . and are left to raise themselves," but in New York parents "tighten the screws, not only on the girls, but on the boys, too" (Glazer and Moynihan 1963: 123). Social workers find that many Puerto Rican boys are disturbed because they are overprotected by parents who have an exaggerated fear of the streets. Parents believe that in New York boys who are given freedom may "find bad friends, may take to drugs, will learn to be disrespectful and disobedient. And even if a boy survives the streets morally, how is he to survive them physically, with cars and trucks whizzing by, and tough Negro and Italian boys ready to beat him up under slight provocation" (Glazer and Moynihan 1963:123).

At adolescence the Puerto Rican boy is expected to become a *macho,* but when he first tries to demonstrate his autonomy, his family may at one moment praise him, and in the next, mock him "almost into insignificance. It is not surprising that a boy caught in this conflict may go to great lengths, even adducing delinquent activities, to avoid ridicule and prove that he is a *macho"* (Minuchin et al. 1967:239).

When parents are unable to cope with rebellious sons, they may report them to social agencies or send them to relatives in Puerto Rico, recall them, and send them back when they again cannot control them. Recent migrants complain that the police in New York prevent parents from disciplining their children in the way they do in Puerto Rico. But the Commonwealth and New York provide about the same degree of legal protection for children, and the parents are rationalizing their inability to adjust to the great freedom American children have.

Dark-skinned Puerto Rican children appear to have the greatest problems. The upward mobility of the family in which children have a wide range of skin color is limited because it is regarded as black. "This family also comes to consider its darker children are Negroes and therefore less favored" (Berle 1958:46), and these children may become the family scapegoats. One social worker noted that "among a group of 20 young Puerto Rican drug addicts, all turned out to be the darkest member of his family" (Berle 1958:49).

In New York the family must assume the controls that are exercised by many communities in Puerto Rico. But because of the way they interact with their children, parents often "release" them to their peer group, and the growing child frequently adopts the values of the gang. However, when the father is absent or fails to measure up to the traditional paternal model, uncles, cousins, and godfathers often become father surrogates, for the Puerto Rican family is more likely to find compensatory male figures than do most black families (Minuchin et al. 1967:236).

Three studies are discussed below to show the impact of child-rearing practices and socioeconomic status on the educational potential and achievement, particularly in language, of Puerto Rican children in New

York. The first study attributes the differences in educational potential between low-income Puerto Ricans and middle-income native-born New Yorkers to the differences in child-rearing practices. However, some of these differences derive from socioeconomic status, for in the second study low-income Puerto Ricans and blacks share some of the traits that differentiate these two groups from the middle class. Finally, the third study, comparing academic achievement of first-grade children among four ethnic groups, both middle and low income, shows the social-class differences in academic ability, but also points to the traditional child-rearing practices in both classes as the primary factor in the "language disability" of Puerto Rican children.

In the study of low-income Puerto Ricans and native-born middle-income New Yorkers, the Puerto Rican fathers had unskilled and semi-skilled jobs; the families were stable and did not live in overcrowded, substandard housing; and the mothers stayed home and took care of their children. The middle-class mothers were found to be businesslike and time-oriented, and the Puerto Rican mothers were person-oriented and not concerned with time. Neither group of mothers pressured the children in feeding, weaning, and toilet training. But the middle-class mothers were actively concerned that their children develop responsibility, independence, task-mastery and verbal ability at an early age, whereas the Puerto Rican mothers did not press their children for achievement in these areas. Thus the middle-class children were verbal and task-oriented, while the Puerto Rican children were very often verbally passive and unresponsive.

The behavioral pattern of the Puerto Rican children does not derive in any way from parental indifference or rejection. Nor does it indicate any inferiority or deficiency in the children. Rather it represents a learned pattern which might be optimal for some other environment but does place the children at a disadvantage in our task-oriented society (Chess et al. 1967:11).

These different cultural patterns, already clearly evident in the behavior of three-year-old children, if continued, "can only result in a much enhanced likelihood for school failure and under-achievement in the Puerto Rican children and for school success in the middle-class children" (Chess et al. 1967:11).

In a comparison between the communication patterns of Puerto Rican and black mothers and their preschool children in a summer Headstart program in New York, the lower-class home and middle-class school settings were found to be congruent in that both require "adaptation to rigid authority structures . . . that tend to reenforce passivity and compliance" (Weissman 1966:88–89). For example, the "command" or directive function of language seemed to be much more meaningful to the lower-class child than the actual content of language. The younger children in both groups, however, were more responsive than the older ones, who were more guarded and impassive.

The Puerto Rican mothers were found to have a *laissez-faire* attitude, which "creates conditions of ambiguity, inconsistency, and lack of a structure in family relationships," that leads "toward passivity and lack of motivation for learning." Nevertheless, the Puerto Rican children were more motivated to master tasks than the black children, and therefore the passivity of the Puerto Rican children was "readily modifiable, reversible and subject to change to more active levels of behavior" (Weissman 1966:82).

The Puerto Rican mothers praised and encouraged their children much more than the black mothers, who were far more directive and critical, and the black children were much more restless and anxious than the Puerto Rican children.

In the home, the Puerto Ricans were more responsive and animated than the blacks and warmer and more hospitable to visitors. The Puerto Rican home was much noisier, "with the mother and father seeming more tolerant or helpless to control very hyperactive play. . . . The Puerto Rican home, even in the face of unemployment, parental confusion and perplexity, seemed to have more hope and optimism" (Weissman 1966:75). The Puerto Ricans showed much greater evidence of extended family relationships. More Puerto Rican fathers were present, helping with household chores and with the children, and joining in the games, particularly with their sons, but when black fathers were present, they tended to remain in the background.

The mothers in both groups not only interacted twice as often with daughters as with sons, but tended to be more warm and playful with daughters. The greater severity and coldness toward the sons seemed to represent displaced or negative reactions "toward the disesteemed or absent male parent," which would "tend to create different attitudes and aptitudes toward achievement" on the part of boys and girls (Weissman 1966:82).

In the study by Lesser, Fifer, and Clark, which sought to determine ethnic and social-class sources of academic abilities, middle- and lower-income Puerto Rican, black, Jewish, and Chinese children in the first grade in the New York City schools were tested on verbal ability, reasoning, numerical facility, and space conceptualization. The test materials were administered in the child's primary language in order to reduce the direct effects of bilingualism upon test scores. The verbal scores of the bilingual Chinese were not significantly higher than those of the Chinese who spoke only English, but "there were too few Puerto Rican children who spoke English only to permit a similar analysis for this group" (1965:72). The Puerto Rican and black children were found to be the most responsive to the testers.

The Jewish girls were superior to the Jewish boys in verbal ability and space conceptualization, but in the other groups the boys achieved higher scores than the girls. The Jewish children in both social classes ranked significantly higher in verbal ability than the other groups, and the blacks and Chinese were significantly higher than the Puerto Ricans. The verbal skills of the Puerto Rican children were the weakest of all their mental abilities and compared unfavorably with the other groups. In the other tests the Puerto Ricans in both classes alternated with the blacks in third and fourth place.

On all tests middle-class children were significantly superior to lower-class children, and the scores of the middle-class children resembled each other to a greater extent than the scores of the lower-class children, but the middle- and lower-class Puerto Ricans were the least widely separated of the four groups (Lesser et al. 1965:60–61).

The findings indicated that social class and ethnicity "do foster the development of a different pattern of abilities, while social-class differences do not modify these basic organizations associated with ethnic-group conditions" (Lesser et al. 1965:82).

The results of the three studies indicate that the language patterns of Puerto Rican children, both in the middle and lower classes, stem primarily from the culture, but in the lower-class Puerto Rican children they are reinforced by patterns common among all low-income ethnic groups. This brings into question the Sapir-Whorf hypothesis, with its claim that world views stem from language patterns.

The verbal patterns of Puerto Rican children, which emphasize *respeto* so heavily, stem from a semifeudal, agricultural society with Latin American values, some of which tend to be liabilities in the work-oriented, industrialized North American society. It is noteworthy that these Latin American values are shared by blue-collar workers in industrialized societies, who also find them to be liabilities.

To the person-oriented Latin American, *personalismo,* the personal connection, is far more important in employment and upward mobility than task mastery. Since lower-class culture is also person-oriented, social class reinforces ethnic values among low-income Puerto Ricans in New York. Latin Americans regard work as a necessary evil, a means to an end, and not a good in itself, and they do not relate task mastery to verbal skills. The upper classes associate such skills with philosophy and poetry, and the lower classes, including those in the

United States, associate them with aggressive verbal exchange, as in the "dirty dozens." When the "command" function of language is more important than the content of language, social class and ethnicity again reinforce each other, for the children of both Puerto Ricans and blue-collar Americans are subject to authoritarian "commands." This lack of emphasis on the content of language, when coupled with the "noise level" of the lower-class home, also retards speech and reading ability, for they hinder the development of auditory discrimination (Leavitt 1962).

Language is a very complex problem for Puerto Ricans in New York. Their ambivalence about race and color is bound up with language, and even very young children are affected. In interviews with first-grade children of different ethnic groups, some of the Puerto Ricans used Spanish to claim membership in "other Latin . . . groups as a source of greater prestige than Puerto Rican identity, while some young Negro children acquire a small Spanish vocabulary and then classify themselves as Puerto Ricans" (Lesser et al. 1965:25).

Since the language of the home is Spanish, a child has little or no knowledge of English when he enters school, unless he has attended a preschool program or a child-care center, or he has an elder sibling or an acculturated relative who speaks English. Migrants are rarely bilingual and are defensive about both Spanish and English. They find that even their language changes in New York, and they must learn many new Spanish words and phrases, derived from English, that are unknown on the island. And learning English is very difficult for people who are barely literate in their own language.

They are expected to have a standard grammatical knowledge of Spanish and a large Spanish vocabulary. Yet they have had almost no schooling and will have learned their tongue largely from illiterate parents and friends. Migrants are expected to try to learn English, but they consider that only children are capable of learning, and that they just cannot (Padilla 1958:66).

Parents rarely train their children purposefully to speak Spanish. "Children are supposed to 'listen to,' rather than 'talk to,' their parents, and the child gets little practice in speaking to them" (Mencher 1958: 233). In the extended family, siblings and adults other than parents teach children to speak, and in the nuclear family, language may be learned even more slowly. Moreover, the good child is the quiet child. Restrictions are placed on his speech, for he must not talk when the father is eating, and must never interrupt or participate in adult conversations. Nevertheless, most children speak a fairly adequate Spanish by the time they are three years old.

Neither language (Spanish) nor play expands the Puerto Rican child's fields of activity and imagination, or helps him solve problems, or broadens his universe. But when he learns English, he acquires a new and important status. He becomes the interpreter and translator for his family and their link with the urban institutions. He gains the approval of his teachers and is more readily accepted by his neighborhood peers, Puerto Rican and non-Puerto Rican.

Between 1960 and 1968 the number of Puerto Ricans born in New York increased from 183,000 to about 250,000 (Hoffman 1968:47, 57). Despite the low socioeconomic status of their parents, racial and ethnic discrimination, problems at home and in school, second-generation Puerto Ricans have made considerable progress. Their achievement is measured not only against the status of their parents, but also against the population of a city which contains about twice as many college graduates per capita as the rest of the country.

The second generation consistently acquired more schooling. Between 1950 and 1960 the number of high school dropouts declined, and the number who graduated from high school and went on to college increased. In 1960 their educational median was 10.3 years for males and 10.8 for females, compared with 12.2 years for persons aged twenty-five to thirty-five on the mainland (Macisco 1968:26). This represented a significant gain over the first generation, especially for the women. But Puerto Ricans still "lag far behind the other-whites in terms of both the percentage of the group in the upper educational categories and the dimension of the shift in these categories" (Kantrowitz 1968:61).

Unemployment declined for the second generation, and once in the labor force they were more likely to be employed than the first generation. The proportions in various occupations had shifted for the second generation by 1960. The number of operatives declined from 40 to 26 percent; and of service workers, from about 18 to 11 percent. The proportion of craftsmen and foremen increased from about 10 to 17 percent; clerical and sales workers, from about 9 to 18 percent; and professional, technical, and executive workers, from about 5.7 to 12.6 percent (Macisco 1968:36). Occupationally the second generation became substantially mobile in the direction of the total United States distribution.

The intergenerational female shift was striking. The percentage of operatives declined from about 66 to 23, and clerical and sales workers increased from about 10 to 43 percent. Puerto Rican second-generation women left the factory for the office. "There is a strong suggestion that the traditionally dominant role [of the male] is being weakend by women's wage earner status. The female is most likely adjusting more effectively to mainland patterns" (Macisco 1968:30). The Puerto Rican women's better adjustment is further confirmed by the fact that they showed only a slight increase in hospital admissions for mental illness in 1967, compared with a substantial increase for the men.

The second generation, however, were still poor in 1960. "Among Puerto Ricans aged 25–34, only 5.7 percent had incomes of at least $6,000 per year as compared with 16.7 percent of the total population" in New York (Kantrowitz 1968:71). But Puerto Ricans were consistent savers as their income rose, and their insolvency declined with length of residence. The Puerto Rican vote rose from about 25,000 in the 1954 election in New York to over 200,000 in 1966 (Senior 1961: 74, 77). Thus, the economic and political acculturation of the younger generation was at least equal to, and in some instances greater than, that of previous immigrants' children.

The rate of intermarriage is of central importance as an index of assimilation, and second-generation Puerto Ricans in New York made significantly more out-group marriages than their parents.

Increases in the rate of out-group marriage among second as compared with first generation Puerto Ricans in 1949 and 1959 were as great as those found by Drachsler for all immigrants in New York, 1908–1912(Fitzpatrick 1966a:395).

More women than men marry out of the group, and may marry out in order to "marry up." Puerto Rican men, on the other hand, "tend to marry women of the same or lower economic status" (Macisco 1968:30).

In 1949 civil marriage was much more common in Puerto Rico than among Puerto Ricans in New York, and Protestant marriages were much more frequent among Puerto Ricans in New York than in Puerto Rico. However, in New York in the period between 1949 and 1959, there was "a strong tendency for Catholic marriages to increase and for Protestant marriages to decrease in the second generation in both 1949 and 1959. This appears to be related to a decline in marriages by Spanish-speaking Pentecostal and Evangelical ministers" (Fitzpatrick (1966a:405–6).

Second-generation Puerto Ricans also marry at a younger age than the first generation, tending toward the young age at marriage which is characteristic of the United States as a whole. The fertility decline of the second generation is also notable. By 1960, "second generation Puerto Ricans have lower fertility than do both the first generation and total United States women." The average number of children for women on the mainland was 2.5; for Puerto Rican women in general, 2.7; for second-generation Puerto Rican women, 2.2 (Macisco 1968:29).

The positive correlation of out-group marriage in the second generation with advance in occupational status, the tendency toward younger age of marriage and the decline of interest in the . . . sects all give evidence of the acceptance of mainland American ways (Fitzpatrick 1966a:406).

Puerto Rican teenagers blend into adolescent American groups, and their speech, clothes, and manners distinguish them from recent migrants. To most of the second generation "home is . . . a New York block," and when they visit the island, they are often "treated and feel like strangers" (Hoffman 1968).

Nevertheless, many second-generation Puerto Ricans experience "a lingering identity crisis" which makes them uncertain whether their values are "urban American or traditionally Latin" (Hoffman 1968). They acknowledge their debt both to the parental and to the New York cultures by referring to themselves as "New Yoricans" (Senior 1968: 77). But they appear to be the only second generation in the United States to have retained their own culture and language, and it is likely that "large segments even of their third generation will remain bilingual and bicultural."

Puerto Rican children switch easily from one idiom to another as they do their homework, talk to parents and friends, and act as interpreters in family dealings with welfare workers and other officials (Hoffman 1968:57).

The ambivalence of the second generation toward American blacks is focused more on a power struggle than on color and race. Blacks are sometimes seen as allies, at other times as rivals. On the one hand, blacks have helped to "politicalize" Puerto Ricans; on the other hand, there is "great, open hostility between Puerto Ricans and Negroes over control of anti-poverty" and school programs. Second-generation Puerto Ricans are frequently militant, "under a young slum-bred leadership," and fight for their rights much more aggressively than the first generation. Among these new leaders "there's practically not one guy who hasn't been in a street gang" (Hoffman 1968:47, 57).

Thirty years ago, when the Puerto Ricans were beginning to migrate in large numbers to the mainland, they might well have been considered "the migrants least likely to succeed."

Nothing—in education, in work experience, work training, or work discipline, in family attitudes, in physical [and mental] health—gave the Puerto Rican migrant an advantage in New York City. Who could have expected to find that the Puerto Rican migration to New York City, then, has been as successful as it has (Glazer and Moynihan 1963:91)?

CHAPTER 11

The Migrants in San Juan and New York:
A Comparison

The values of the culture of poverty transcend differences between rural and urban areas, and also between nations. Thus the slums of San Juan and New York share many attitudes and behavior patterns. Aside from climate and language, the differences between the two areas stem from the varying dominant values of the island and the mainland, and from the varying socioeconomic factors in a small, poor, industrializing country and one of the most highly industrialized and affluent nations in the world.

Occupations, Income, and Consumer Practices

In 1951 agricultural workers in Puerto Rico earned, on the average, $6.50 a week (Friedlander 1965:121) and were unemployed for several months of the year. Because of their limited skills and education they had the least chance for upward mobility when they migrated to San Juan or New York.

In San Juan the rural migrants constitute the vast majority of the lowest socioeconomic stratum. In 1960 a small number were pushcart peddlers and owned tiny stores, 1 percent were lower white-collar workers, 16 percent were skilled workers, and 77 percent had semi-skilled and unskilled jobs. About 73 percent worked full time; the rest were unemployed and subemployed (Rogler and Hollingshead 1965:48).

In the same period in New York 5.5 percent of the Puerto Ricans had upper white-collar jobs, 11.5 percent were lower white-collar workers, 10.5 percent were skilled workers, and two-thirds did semiskilled and unskilled work. In 1966, 85 percent of the Puerto Ricans in New

York lived in poverty areas; 10 percent were unemployed and about 33 percent were underemployed.[1]

Although many more women work outside the home in San Juan than in the rural areas, in 1960 only 22 percent of the labor force in Puerto Rico was female, compared with about 39 percent of the Puerto Rican-born labor force in the United States (Macisco 1968:35). In Puerto Rico most of the women workers were in the low-job category. The men outnumbered the women at the high level by about 5.5 to 1; at the medium level, by about 24 to 1; and at the low level, by only 3 to 1 (Tumin and Feldman 1961:328–329). In New York, Puerto Rican women slightly outnumbered the men in the low-level jobs, and almost equaled them in the medium and upper-level jobs. Almost 4 percent of the women had upper white-collar employment, 15 percent had lower white-collar jobs, and about 73 percent were operatives and service workers.[2]

In 1959 the median family income of Class V, the lowest socioeconomic stratum, comprising 67 percent of the total San Juan population, was about $1,350, and for Class IV members, comprising 20 percent of the population, it was about $2,550 (Rogler and Hollingshead 1965:51). In New York in 1959 about 34 percent of the Puerto Rican families had an income under $3,000; and 54 percent had an income from $3,000 to $7,000.[3]

Puerto Ricans with the darkest skins are preponderantly in the lowest classes in Puerto Rico, as well as on the mainland, for economic discrimination against blacks is by far the most frequently cited type of discrimination in Puerto Rico (Tumin and Feldman 1961:239). In fact, the poor in San Juan refer to the middle and upper classes as "the whites," and to themselves as "the darker ones" (Rogler and Hollingshead 1965:63).

In December, 1968, aid to dependent children averaged $6.95 a month per child in Puerto Rico, compared with $89.44 a month per child in New York (Kihss 1969:38). In the early 1960s, about half the families in New York receiving supplementary aid were Puerto Rican, and a third of the Puerto Rican children in the city received aid (Glazer and Moynihan 1963:118). Children on welfare are more retarded in school and grow up with the values of the culture of unemployment, but because they receive considerably more welfare assistance in New

---

[1]U.S. Department of Labor, *Labor Force Experience of the Puerto Rican Worker, op. cit.,* pp. 17, 26.

[2]*Ibid.,* p. 17.

[3]*Ibid.,* p. 21.

York, migrants do not shift their children to relatives and friends nearly as often as they do in Puerto Rico.

In 1960, making allowances for differences in cost of living, "the typical Puerto Rican could expect to double his income by moving to the continent . . . with movement from rural sections of the island to urban centers on the continent bringing maximum gain" (Gray 1962:187).

In Puerto Rico the rank-and-file union membership is generally apathetic because, as Gordon Lewis (1963:229) points out, most unions are controlled by unscrupulous labor lawyers and corrupt politicians, and mainland-based national unions may negotiate with employers without consulting the locals on the island. Also, mainland-owned plants, established in Puerto Rico because of tax exemptions and low wages, threaten closure when unions become militant. In the last few years unions have begun to "Puertoricanize," but in the face of high, chronic unemployment, Class V members are still relatively powerless, and the traditional employer-employee relationships prevail, requiring deference and submissiveness from employees.

In the United States, the working classes learned to "talk back" early in the history of the nation, and this attitude has been reinforced by the growth and strength of labor unions, particularly since the 1930s. In New York, about 60 percent of the Puerto Ricans belong to unions, and although some unions are racketeering and bureaucratic, New York is a "union town." In the militant new unions that are organizing low-level workers, Puerto Ricans have risen rapidly to leadership and have then become active in politics. When the Puerto Rican migrant engages in union and political activities in New York, he emerges from the culture of poverty, which is much smaller, proportionately, on the mainland than on the island. In San Juan, the migrant is generally isolated from the major social institutions, and escapes from the culture of poverty in the relatively rare instances when he lives in a cohesive, integrated neighborhood or is upwardly mobile.

Consumer practices among the lower and middle classes in both Puerto Rico and the mainland are based on installment buying, but because of the person-orientation of the working class, which is culturally reinforced among the Puerto Ricans, the migrants become involved with local stores that have a very high mark-up, keep debtors in economic bondage, and intensify economic insecurity and anxieties. But as length of residence in New York increases and income rises, Puerto Ricans adopt the value of thrift which is more characteristic of the stable blue-collar workers, and consistently become more solvent. In San Juan, as in the rural areas, the migrant has little incentive to be thrifty. With a much lower income and much less possibility of upward mobility, he has little opportunity to structure his economic life.

Housing and Neighborhood Life

In 1960, about three-fourths of the migrants in San Juan lived in shanties, tenements, and low-cost public housing, but more than twice as many lived in shanties as in tenements. The tenements and housing projects correspond in most respects to those in New York, but in New York there is no counterpart of the San Juan shantytowns, which form the bulk of the slums in the city.

Shantytowns are built on marginal land unfit for commercial or residential use. The largest shantytown is located on swampy land adjoining a channel which was for many years the principal sewer of San Juan. Built of scrap material by unskilled labor, the shanty corresponds to the rural hut. As land becomes scarce, the shanties are built on long piles over the swamps and open water, and are often flooded during storms. Since garbage was not collected in the shantytowns up through the early 1960s, garbage thrown under the houses became a solid base in time. Shantytowns had no sewer pipes or cesspools, and toilets emptied into open ditches running from the houses to the alleys.

In the 1950s, the government began to provide the shantytowns with street lighting and wooden sidewalks, water pipes and public faucets, health and welfare services, police and fire protection, and elementary schools. But in 1960 the shantytowns still had the highest inicidence of infant mortality, tuberculosis, and pneumonia in the San Juan area. No more than a foot or two of land separates adjacent shanties, the majority of which have only one bedroom, with as many as three to five children per bed.

More shanties are owned by the residents who pay no rent and therefore resist moving into housing projects. The range of income is much greater in a shantytown than in a housing project, which admits and retains only those with limited incomes, and has proportionately more residents on welfare. Some studies describe the shantytown as better integrated, with fewer fatherless families and less delinquency, because the father has more authority and autonomy than in the project, and residents exercise greater controls over the community. Neighborhood integration is also correlated with bedroom density and the quantity and quality of neighborhood improvements and nuisances, and some projects are also well integrated. Neighborhood integration tends to rise with higher income and education, the "right color," church attendance, and participaton in voluntary organizations.

In the shantytown, the migrant retains his folk culture and may raise pigs, chickens, and plants. Real urbanization begins when he lives in a tenement or housing project in San Juan. In New York his urbanization begins immediately, usually with residence in a tenement. Living conditions in the San Juan shantytowns are generally far worse in terms of health and comfort than in the most dilapidated New York tenement, and "for an unemployed canecutter a dismal New York tenement may represent a ticket in the lottery of a more abundant life" (Berle 1958:61).

About 21 percent of Class V members in San Juan and 15 percent of Puerto Ricans in New York live in housing projects, where health improves considerably, especially for the children. In New York there are more than fourteen times as many applications for the projects as there are vacancies. Public housing in New York destroyed cohesive ethnic communities and going businesses, substituted uniform "high rises" for architectural diversity, evolved a powerful youth subculture, and helped drive the white middle class to the suburbs. But it also brought parks and community centers, far greater integration of ethnic groups than exists in private housing, and a degree of stability into the slums. Few people move from project apartments, for no better housing can be obtained in either San Juan or New York for the money.

When the migrant arrives in San Juan, he stays with relatives who help him find a job and a place to live. In New York the extended family is less important, and while fewer older migrants turn away a jobless and homeless kinsman, Puerto Ricans brought up in New York seldom recognize obligations toward recent migrants. However, the Migration Division of the Commonwealth Labor Department, as well as mainland agencies, churches, and hometown associations help them find employment and orient them to the city. But such extensive paternalistic assistance may also retard the formation of a strong ethnic community.

In New York the Puerto Rican ethnic community has been largely dispersed by slum clearance, urban redevelopment, and a serious housing shortage. The remaining concentrations are in mixed slums where interethnic hostility is intense and overt. Although neighbors help each other in emergencies, relations with neighbors tend to be ridden by conflict among the poor, for few neighborhoods in the culture of poverty are cohesive and socially integrated. While there is considerable delinquency in the San Juan slums, in the New York slums fear of the streets is pervasive, especially among the migrants, who keep the children indoors all day long, summer and winter. At the same time, close personal interethnic friendships are formed, and the common struggle for better housing and schools encourages interethnic cooperation and alliances.

The American demand for rapid acculturation makes migration to New York far more stressful than to San Juan. In New York, the assault on Puerto Rican identity, weak to start with, leads the migrant to accept the dominant denigratory valuation of his culture and racial mixture. Thus, if he is dark-skinned he may deny his identity and take refuge in Spanish credentials, or if he is white and speaks English without an accent, he may deny his language and origins. The intermediately colored Puerto Rican in New York is the classical marginal man, for he is identified as black despite his denial. Although the Puerto Rican black in San Juan encounters discrimination in housing and employment, in New York he faces hostility both as a Puerto Rican and as a black.

The Puerto Rican who assimilates into the American black subculture, however, may for the first time openly acknowledge his negritude, for in Puerto Rico few people identify as black or want to be so identified. Also, New York politics sanctifies ethnicity and has historically encouraged interethnic accommodation. The Protestant churches also help to organize grass-roots interethnic political, social, and economic programs in the slums. As they are "politicalized" in the struggle for their rights as a bilingual and bicultural group, it is in New York that Puerto Ricans finally appear to be gaining a strong ethnic identity.

Religion

Nominally Catholic, the Puerto Rican lower classes have weak ties with the Church both on the island and the mainland. The Catholic Church is inconspicuous in the slums of San Juan, and in New York the absence of a parish with Puerto Rican Spanish-speaking priests has prevented positive identification with Catholicism. Thus the Church has failed to provide the migrants with the community they badly need. Judging by the increase of Catholic marriages in New York, however, the second generation appears to be turning to the traditional faith as part of the process of "Americanization." Devotion to the saints and the Virgin is widespread in both cities, and baptism and *compadrazgo* persist as the principal religious rituals.

A substantial minority of Puerto Ricans are zealous Protestants in New York and many Protestant churches have Puerto Rican ministers who conduct services in Spanish. Church-related Catholic and Protestant organizations appear to help the migrants far more in New York than in San Juan, and the clergy has also organized grass-roots groups for community action in New York.

In both San Juan and New York, the revivalist sects and the Spiritualist mediums provide extremely important help in conjugal and intergenerational conflict, and for people who are emotionally disturbed. In New York, they also offer the migrants a tight community, as well as a link with the island, and in San Juan, they are among the few sources of social support outside of the nuclear and extended families.

Health

An important reason for migration to New York is its superior health facility, for many of the migrants suffer from poor health. The San Juan slums have a high incidence of infant mortality, tuberculosis, pneumonia, diarrhea, anemia, and intestinal parasites, the principal causes of illness being malnutrition, undernourishment, and unfavorable living conditions. In New York, the migrants have a high accident rate during their first year in the city, and a high rate of hospital admissions for mental illness, tuberculosis, pertussis, and, especially for children, major respiratory infections. Only a limited number of migrants live in the housing projects in San Juan and New York, where health improves markedly.

Since public health personnel in the insular rural areas seldom bother to explain the causes of illness or death to the *jíbaros,* the older migrants in both cities retain their folk medical beliefs and practices. To deal with illness the migrants try home remedies first and then visit public clinics and hospitals. If scientific medicine does not work, they frequently go to a Spiritualist medium, for many believe that illness is caused by the witchcraft of envious people. Even Puerto Ricans born and raised in New York sometimes consult a Spiritualist.

The migrants rarely practice preventive health measures, although they are widely advertised in New York. The modest Puerto Rican woman is reluctant to undergo a physical examination, and most blue-collar workers are not future-oriented. In addition, the migrant, sensitized by his previous negative experience in the rural public health centers and hospitals, tends to avoid unfriendly or patronizing agencies. Frequently New York medical personnel and Puerto Ricans are frustrated because they operate from different cultural premises. However, the migrants cooperate when they are certain of personal interest and continuity of treatment.

Illness is an important mechanism for reestablishing ties that have been broken between relatives and friends, and also for eliciting compassion and help from members of ethnic groups in New York who are usually hostile to one another. Illness also has a profound impact on the everyday life of the migrant. In both cities the sick husband feels very threatened when his wife takes over his wage-earning role. When the wife is ill, relatives assume her functions in San Juan, but in New York the extended family may be absent or dispersed, and the husband who is forced to take care of the household and children may modify his view of male and female roles.

Oscar Lewis found that many of the migrants in the San Juan slums had a history of psychopathology going back for several generations, and everywhere schizophrenia seems to be disproportionately concentrated in the low socioeconomic strata. Based on an estimate of 10,000 schizophrenics, a rate of 435 psychotics per 100,000 population is indicated for Puerto Rico as a whole (Fitzpatrick and Gould 1968:31). The vast majority of schizophrenics live with their families, for public psychiatric facilities in Puerto Rico are very limited. Puerto Ricans are generally horrified by psychopathology, and the lower classes in both the rural and urban areas also ridicule the *loco* and stigmatize those who are treated professionally.

In New York for the period 1948–1951, the rate of schizophrenia for male Puerto Ricans was twice that of the total male rate, and the Puerto Rican female rate was about one and a half times greater than the total female rate. The hospital admissions data for mental illness in 1967 showed only a slight increase for Puerto Rican women, but a significant increase for the men along with a much higher incidence of alcoholic psychoses. On the basis of an estimated Puerto Rican population of 909,500 in New York City in 1967,[4] and the total admissions rate of 2,903 for Puerto Ricans in 1967, (Fitzpatrick and Gould 1968: 50), the rate of Puerto Rican psychotics in the metropolitan area was about 320 per 100,000, compared with 435 in Puerto Rico.

Most schizophrenics on the mainland are placed in public mental hospitals, where they occupy one-fourth of the beds (Rogler and Hollingshead 1965:6). When Puerto Rican psychotics are placed in institutions, however, their condition may worsen. Prolonged separation from the family, which exhibits a remarkable strength in coping with mental disturbance, is a source of considerable stress to Puerto Ricans. The emphasis on the confinement of Puerto Rican psychotics may be due to the lack of Spanish-speaking staff in the great majority of the hospitals serving Spanish-speaking neighborhoods in New York. For example, the *ataque,* called the "Puerto Rican Syndrome," a cultural

---

[4]Personal communication, Commonwealth of Puerto Rico, Department of Labor, Migration Division, April 14, 1969.

reaction to catastrophe that is widespread among lower-income Puerto Ricans on both the island and the mainland, may be misdiagnosed as a more serious personality disorder by those unfamiliar with the language and the culture. Also, very few Spanish-speaking psychiatrists are employed in the Bureau for Child Guidance of the Board of Education, although in 1967, with a Puerto Rican enrollment of 22.1 percent in the schools, 33 percent of the children in the "special schools" for behavior problems were Puerto Rican.

Mental health practitioners severely criticize those of their colleagues who often unwittingly promulgate the middle-class Protestant ethic under the guise of science, and who use their power to confine powerless people of other ethnic groups and social classes, whom they neither like nor understand. However, New York City is building community health centers, and several hospitals in areas with large Puerto Rican populations are now treating patients in the context of their family and sociocultural milieu, and relating mental health problems to poverty, cognitive deficits, migration, and the tensions of changing neighborhoods. Lincoln Hospital in the Bronx has identified the strengths of Puerto Ricans in the capacity of the family to manage emotional disturbances, in the hometown associations, and in the Pentecostal churches and Spiritualism.

Thus, despite the many disadvantages that confront mentally ill Puerto Ricans, New York City also has facilities and methods of treatment that San Juan cannot afford, and the rate of mental illness of Puerto Ricans in New York appears to be much lower than in Puerto Rico.

Marriage and the Family

As the traditional society modernizes, the extended family usually changes to the nuclear form. But in a stratified society, the various classes experience social change, including changes in the family, differently.

Although the nuclear family has made inroads in the middle class and some of the rural subcultures, throughout Puerto Rico the institution of the extended family is still very strong, particularly among the rural and urban poor who remain outside of the economic mainstream. In the United States, where the nuclear family predominates, the extended family also persists among blue-collar workers because it performs the same functions as in Puerto Rico. It provides stability in the face of economic insecurity, even though the insecurity is much less extensive and profound on the mainland.

Paradoxically, in the modern urban milieu of New York it is the extended family among the Puerto Rican migrants that accommodates most easily to change and is most upwardly mobile, while the migrants who are compelled to acculturate from a nuclear family base are the least mobile and the most resistant to change. In San Juan the extended family is one of the few certain sources of support for the low-income person, but in New York it is often absent or dispersed, and the acculturating nuclear family suffers great stress in the ethnically mixed slums, where it is often isolated even from other Puerto Ricans.

Where the extended family persists, ties between its members are strengthened by ritual kinship, especially for women without husbands, who leave their children with kin-godparents in Puerto Rico or New York as they travel back and forth in search of work or a new life.

Polygyny and free multiple unions have always been widespread in rural Puerto Rico, among the rich and the poor alike, and in the early 1950s more than a third of those with up to four years of schooling were living in consensual union on the island. The consensual union and its offspring are accepted in the slum subcultures in both San Juan and New York, but are condemned by middle-class Puerto Ricans and the larger mainland society. On the mainland, however, it appears that very many Puerto Ricans adopt the dominant American value of legal marriage, for the rate of consensual unions among migrants who return to the island is less than half the rate in Puerto Rico. At the same time the rate of illegitimacy among Puerto Ricans in New York doubled between 1957 and 1967, along with a significant rise in illegitimacy among blacks and whites, indicating a general growing rejection of legal marriage as the socializing institution. Migrants often become "loose and lost" in New York, but prostitution appears to be less extensive than in San Juan because women have greater economic resources.

The ideal of the small family prevails among Puerto Ricans everywhere but, principally because of the communication barrier between husband and wife, especially in matters of sex, the lower-class Puerto Rican family remains large, and in New York it is significantly larger than the non-Puerto Rican family. Low-income Puerto Ricans both in San Juan and New York rely extensively on sterilization to arrest family growth, but the operation is generally performed after the family is already larger than desired by either spouse. The large family is more typically broken, on relief, lives in substandard housing, and the children particularly experience more illness.

Puerto Ricans brought up in New York reject sterilization as a means of contraception. And the fertility rate of second-generation Puerto Ricans in New York is lower not only than that of their parents, but also than the average on the mainland. The children of the migrants in

San Juan also have smaller families as they move into the middle class.

Only over his wife and children is the lower-class Puerto Rican man able to exercise power and authority, the essence of masculinity both in North America and Latin America. But male authority rests on the ability to support the family, and this the migrants find very difficult to do. In San Juan many more women work outside the home than in the rural areas, while the man is almost as insecure economically as in the rural areas. The women become less willing to accept their subordinate role and particularly resent male philandering, which is as great as in previous generations. Marital relations deteriorate, physical violence between husband and wife increases, and frequently the matrifocal family emerges. In fact, in the San Juan slums the women are more aggressive than the men, and it is the man who often tries to prevent the break-up of the family. The study of schizophrenia in San Juan, by Rogler and Hollingshead (1965), clearly demonstrates that the migrants find the traditional sex roles onerous and dysfunctional in an industrial society where they are under great stress, but do not know how to modify them or adopt alternative roles.

Almost twice as many Puerto Rican women are in the labor force on the mainland as on the island, and in New York their economic independence, which is much greater than in San Juan, is considerably increased by the substantially higher welfare assistance. In New York the male migrant feels doubly threatened because he has increased difficulty in getting a job as automation accelerates, manufacturing declines and educational requirements for employment are upgraded.

The link between male autonomy and dependency is pronounced in the culture of poverty both on the island and the mainland. The Puerto Rican man is dependent on women from his earliest days, and he leaves all practical matters to his wife. Although the American family is also patriarchal, sex roles are less sharply segregated, and marital relationships are more egalitarian, even among the working classes, than in Puerto Rico. With this model, the Puerto Rican wife not only flouts her subordinate role, but presses strongly for role desegregation. Role segregation is maintained in San Juan because the woman can count on the help of members of the extended family, but in New York, where relatives may be dispersed or absent, the Puerto Rican working wife insists that her husband share household and child-rearing chores, problems, and recreation.

In the New York slum subculture, as well as in the rural areas of the island and in San Juan, masculinity is expressed by sexual adventurism, drinking, and gambling. The male migrant increases the activities when he cannot provide for the family, and his wife becomes insubordinate.

The Puerto Rican woman regards her husband as exploitative, irresponsible, and lacking in respect for her, and wavers between leaving him and preserving the family.

Between 1951 and 1967, schizophrenia among Puerto Rican women in New York rose only slightly, but the significant rise in schizophrenia and alcoholic psychoses among Puerto Rican men testifies to their unsatisfactory socioeconomic status, lack of social recognition and participation, and poor integration into the family. Nevertheless, even among disorganized Puerto Rican families in New York sex roles are more stable than among blacks. Puerto Rican women regard the husband as integral to the family and often suppress their desire for greater equality and freedom in order to support the culturally induced male need for dominance. The woman's attitude may also stem from the fact that in New York the nuclear family is often isolated, and the woman has fewer relatives on whom to depend than in San Juan.

Both in San Juan and New York the extended family, the revivalist sects, and the Spiritualist mediums help to solve family problems among the Puerto Rican migrants. And as the Puerto Rican man gradually acculturates to mainland norms, he is regarded as a potentially good husband. He learns to feel less threatened when his wife works outside the home and makes a financial contribution. He helps with child rearing and with household chores, does not "run around" as much with other women, he and his wife share problems and recreation, and he becomes more deeply committed to his family. Sexual role desegregation accelerates with upward mobility, for middle-class models are more clearly egalitarian than those of blue-collar workers. Nevertheless, even the acculturated Puerto Rican man subscribes to the traditional values about women's role and prefers to marry recent migrants rather than Puerto Rican women reared in New York. The women, on the other hand, tend to marry "up and out."

Roles also change in San Juan, but far more slowly because the traditional patriarchal family is still the ideal among the lower classes, and the rural migrant has less opportunity for upward mobility into the middle class.

Child Rearing

Child-rearing practices are influenced by the structure and status of the family within the context of dominant values. But above all, the city itself, whether San Juan or New York, imposes its own distinct changes and problems.

Between 1946 and 1958 the number of babies delivered in hospitals in Puerto Rico rose from 16 to 66 percent, and in the latter part of this period women began to visit clinics for prenatal care and immunizations for children. Migrants who began childbearing in Puerto Rico during the last decade increased their use of professional services as they continued to bear children in New York. Those who bear all their children in New York generally make maximum use of free clinics and hospitals.

In the San Juan shantytowns, migrant women continue the rural custom of breast-feeding until the next pregnancy, but they may also use supplementary bottles. Since in New York many more Puerto Rican women work outside the home, exclusive bottle-feeding is very widespread, permitting the use of mother surrogates. Children continue to feed from bottles until they enter school and even after, and also use pacifiers extensively. Thus oral dependency is prolonged long after the usual period on the mainland. Eating and sleeping are unscheduled, and in neither city is the lower-class Puerto Rican child trained for a time-oriented industrial society.

When the family already has two or three children, the mother directs her resentment over each successive pregnancy at her husband and children. In the extended family, "significant others" are sources of comfort to the children. However, when the new baby arrives it is accepted warmly and its every desire is indulged, except in the nuclear family in New York, where the mother may have no one to help her.

Both in San Juan and New York childhood starts abruptly when the baby begins to walk or another child is born. In New York, toilet training is harsh, is frequently followed by long-lasting enuresis, and seems to be associated with the frustrations and discomforts of tenement living. In the project apartment, with its private bathroom and greater conveniences, toilet training is more permissive. The recent migrant does not use diapers on the baby, except when he is consciously imitating the middle class in San Juan, or when he has accepted American standards of modesty and hygiene in New York. In fact, severe toilet training may also be a reaction to the disgust expressed by Americans over feces dropped anywhere in the house by babies without diapers.

Wherever housing is overcrowded and children must sleep in the parents' room, the child is aware of parental sexual relations at an early age. Because of the fear of incest the modesty training of girls starts very early, but among the more acculturated Puerto Ricans in New York modesty training becomes less restrictive for the girl and more restrictive for the boy. In New York the girl's diaper may be changed by the father or an uncle, but this never occurs in San Juan.

The practice of fondling the young boy's bare genitals to encourage *machismo* is still traditional in the San Juan slums, but is declining in New York, where the boy is now covered more often. The rate of gastrointestinal infection caused by the fecal contamination of objects is therefore also decreasing in New York.

The principal value by which the Puerto Rican child is enculturated is respect. In some of the rural subcultures respect is taught by precept and example, but in San Juan and New York it can be enforced only by physical punishment, which is usually violent and capricious, particularly for boys. In New York the children who are punished the most severely are those in the isolated, tradition-bound, nuclear family with the least status. The acculturated and socially mobile families, where both parents are working and the wife can depend on the help of her husband and other relatives, rely least on physical punishment and most on verbal guidance.

Aggression is regarded as most threatening to respect. Yet, because of the increased conflicts between parents and between parents and children, and the model of physical violence in the streets, even very young children in the San Juan slums are more aggressive than children in any other subculture or class, and parents permit more aggression against themselves. In New York parents are embarrassed and angered by a child's aggression which, they believe, creates a bad impression on Americans. Children are also much more restricted and dependent in New York because recent migrants are very much afraid of the violence and aggression of the slum streets. But acculturated parents are less protective of their children, allow them to play more freely in the streets, and also permit some aggression against themselves.

In New York the discontinuities in child rearing are sharper than in San Juan. In the traditional Puerto Rican family boys are more indulged than girls in infancy and early childhood, but they are also punished more severely, especially by the mother, for a show of aggression. The boy dichotomizes his responses to the conflicting demands of the home and the community. He suppresses aggression at home and acts it out excessively in school and in the neighborhood.

In the slums of San Juan and New York boys have far fewer responsibilities and much less contact with the father than in the rural areas. Paternal authority decreases as the man becomes more marginal to the family, and the authority of the peer group becomes primary, especially in the projects where the youth subculture is often very powerful. If the father is absent or unable to exert his authority, an uncle or a godfather may become a father surrogate, even in New York, and some controls are maintained over the children.

In San Juan the adolescent boy comes and goes freely and has no difficulty achieving *machismo*. But in New York, where he is far more protected and restricted, he may overreact and become delinquent in the effort to prove his masculinity. In attempts at control parents may report a son to the official agencies, send him to relatives in Puerto Rico, recall him, and send him back again. In the family with a wide color range the children who are most often rejected both in San Juan and New York are those with the darkest skin. In New York they may also become the scapegoat if the family does not succeed in moving upward, and those who are very dark-skinned are the most likely to become drug addicts.

Girls are guarded in both San Juan and New York, and are expected to stay close to the home, but in the city play activities are less segregated by sex, and young people are able to meet outside of the neighborhood. Although they still internalize the ideal of virginity, many girls start married life with a consensual union. In New York parents are extremely confused by the many different models of child rearing and adolescent behavior. The coeducational activities of the churches and the settlement houses, where boys and girls are taught to relate to each other less exploitatively and not exclusively on a sexual basis, are particularly threatening to the rural migrants, who view them as a prelude to pregnancy.

At adolescence, the girls are expected to become proper *señoritas,* but in New York they strenuously resist the traditional restrictions as they see the independence of girls in other ethnic groups. Parents say the authorities prevent them from disciplining their children in the traditional way, but in fact they are helpless in the face of the great freedom of American children. Moreover, the roles of *macho* and *señorita* become somewhat blurred in New York, where adolescents of both sexes are attending high school and preparing for skilled jobs. In San Juan adolescents are usually working for a living and the girls are preparing to function in their primary biological role.

Eventually the more acculturated migrants tend to reject the view that the child is *sin capacidad,* and stereotypes of the aggressive boy and the passive girl give way to the belief that "children are all the same." Affection and punishment tend to become equalized, the father becoming less distant and the mother less authoritarian with boys. Parents buy toys and books to advance the development of the preschool child and become involved with their children's play. They no longer demand instant obedience and are more tolerant of the child's impulses and desires.

In fact, the acculturating Puerto Rican family in New York veers in the direction of the middle-class mainland family, where "the child is seen as the adult's partner" rather than as his inferior, and each individual regulates the family "for self rather than family preservation." Only in the American context of child rearing "does the individual ego receive so much opportunity and recognition." (Maier 1965:71).

In their conflicts with their parents Puerto Rican children are struggling to achieve the ego development and freedom of American children. But in San Juan the conflicts between parents and children, like those between husbands and wives, tend to remain unresolved because the principal role models are still traditional. Although these models are dysfunctional, there is no clear reason for rapid change to more functional roles since the majority of the migrants and their children have little opportunity for upward mobility. Thus the changes in child rearing that occur in New York with acculturation and upward mobility take place far more gradually or not at all in the slums of San Juan.

The Second Generation: Education and Upward Mobility

In 1940, only 51 percent of the school-age population in Puerto Rico attended school, and half the parents of the adult migrants had less than a year of schooling.[5] The adult migrants achieved more education. In 1960 in San Juan, 64 percent of Class V members had 0–4 years of school; 28 percent, 5–8 years; and 8 percent, 9–12 years (Rogler and Hollingshead 1965:49). The median education for Class V members was three years, compared with 7.9 years for San Juan as a whole (Caplow et al. 1964:125). In 1960 in New York City, 70 percent of the Puerto Ricans twenty-five years old or more had completed 0–8 years of school, compared with 40 percent of "other whites" and about 45 percent of nonwhites; 17 percent of the Puerto Ricans had completed 8 years; and 27 percent, 9–12 years.[6] Puerto Ricans had the lowest level of formal education in New York City in 1960, but the median education for persons twenty-five years old or more in Puerto Rico was 4.6 years, compared with 8.0 years for the Puerto Rican-born male on the mainland, and 7.2 years for the female (Macisco 1968:35).

The turning point in parental expectations for children's education

---

[5]Commonwealth of Puerto Rico, *A Summary in Facts & Figures, op. cit.,* p. 6.
[6]U.S. Department of Labor, *op. cit.,* p. 20.

in Puerto Rico comes when parents have themselves had more than four years of school. But in the late 1950s, only 36 percent of Class V members had five or more years of schooling. Two-thirds of the children of Class V members were below their chronological age in grade placement, the boys almost two years and the girls, almost three. "If one is lucky, he finishes the sixth grade" (Rogler and Hollingshead 1965:63), and in the San Juan slums, elementary school graduation is an event to be celebrated. However, six years is about twice the amount of schooling the adult migrants achieved.

A high school education is essential for movement into the white-collar class, but in the early 1960s, 66 percent of the boys between ages fourteen and nineteen were school drop-outs and about 20 percent of all those fourteen years of age or over were illiterate (O. Lewis 1965:xxxvi). Although the female adult migrant receives less education than the male in the rural areas, the number of male drop-outs exceeded the number of female drop-outs in San Juan in the middle 1960s.

In the dual educational system of San Juan the poor children attend the public schools and the vast majority of middle- and upper-class children attend private and parochial schools. This has led to the demand that the private schools be abolished as "an instrument of social, economic, racial and religious discrimination" (G. Lewis 1963: 464). With every increase in years of school completed, the proportion of white children becomes greater compared with mulattoes and especially blacks (Tumin and Feldman 1961:229).

In New York about 85 percent of the Puerto Ricans live in poverty areas where most of the elementary schools are residentially segregated and teacher and pupil turnover is very high. Special programs and compensatory education have so far proved ineffective in raising the academic performance of Puerto Rican children, which is considerably below national norms. New York City has instituted bilingual programs to help Spanish-speaking children learn English more easily only so that they may acculturate more rapidly to the mainland. Despite the demands of the Puerto Rican community, the schools are reluctant to promote bilingualism and biculturalism as values in themselves.

English is taught as a second language in the Puerto Rican public schools, but the children have little incentive to learn it, and most migrants are not bilingual. In New York, however, learning English raises the Puerto Rican child's normally low status in the family when he serves as its interpreter with the official agencies, increases his acceptance by his peers, and gains the approval of the school.

The minimum legal school-leaving age, enforced in New York, is sixteen years. In Puerto Rico it is seventeen years, but the law is not

enforced.[7] Despite the high drop-out rate in some of the heavily-popu-
lated Puerto Rican sections of New York, many Puerto Rican children
manage to complete high school, particularly vocational high school.
In 1960 the educational median for second-generation Puerto Ricans
was 10.3 years for males and 10.8 years for females, compared with
12.2 years for all persons aged twenty-five to thirty-four years on the
mainland (Macisco 1968:26). This represented a significant gain over
the first generation, particularly for the women. Although Puerto Ricans
still lag considerably behind "other whites" and blacks in the City
University enrollment, their enrollment in the community colleges increased substantially when open enrollment was instituted in 1970.

In both San Juan and New York the migrants find it difficult to
implement their educational aspirations for their children, and middle-
class teachers are generally not well trained to educate lower-class
children. In San Juan, however, the migrant wants his children to complete elementary school, and in New York he wants them to complete
high school, and the children, especially the girls, increasingly live up
to parental expectations.

Every educational step upward is accompanied by an increase in
income—the most disproportionate income gain in San Juan occurs in
the transition from 1–4 to 5–8 years of education (Tumin and Feldman
1961:229). Most of the children of the migrants in San Juan are in the
5–8 group. In 1960, 11 percent of this group were in Class III, consisting mainly of clerical and sales workers, with a median per capita
income of $1,350; 56 percent were in Class IV, consisting mainly of
skilled workers, with a median per capita income of about $575; and
28 percent were in Class V, consisting of semiskilled and unskilled
workers, with a median per capita income of $260 (Rogler and Hollings-
head 1965:51). Classes III and IV are much more employed than Class V.

For second-generation Puerto Ricans in New York unemployment
also declined, and once in the labor force they are more likely to be
employed than the first generation. Among second-generation Puerto
Ricans 25–34 years of age in 1960, 16.7 percent of the men and 11.7
percent of the women were in professional, technical, and executive
positions; about 17 percent of the men and 46 percent of the women
were in clerical and sales work; 18 percent of the men and about 2
percent of the women were skilled workers; 37 percent of the men and
36 percent of the women were operatives and service workers. The
women made much greater gains than the men in the middle range, and

---

[7]Personal communication, Commonwealth of Puerto Rico, Migration Division,
April 16, 1969.

the men made somewhat more gains than the women in the upper range. The median per capita income for second-generation males was $4,125 and for females, $2,430, compared with $3,053 and $2,034 for first-generation males and females, and with $4,823 and $1,848 for the total male and female population in the United States aged 25–34 years in 1960 (Macisco 1968:35–37).

This means that second-generation Puerto Ricans were still poor in 1960. Only 5.7 percent had annual incomes of at least $6,000, compared with 16.7 percent of the total New York population (Kantrowitz 1968:71). But their upward mobility was much greater than that of the children of the migrants in San Juan.

The second-generation Puerto Ricans in New York appear to have made as much economic progress as the children of previous immigrants. Politically they have made even more progress, under a slum-bred leadership. They have acculturated in speech, clothes and manners; they have intermarried at the same rate as previous immigrants; their fertility is lower not only than that of their parents, but also than the average on the mainland; and they appear to be turning to the traditional religion and away from the sects.

But unlike the children of previous immigrants, they remain bilingual and bicultural, and are perhaps the first group of second-generation Americans to practice cultural pluralism. Many white Puerto Ricans acknowledge their origins with pride, and many dark-skinned Puerto Ricans are for the first time identifying themselves as blacks. It is in New York that the Puerto Ricans finally seem to be gaining a strong sense of their own ethnic and racial identity.

PART IV

STUTTERING AND STRESSES

CHAPTER 12

Stuttering and Stresses

I hypothesized that stuttering incidence would be higher among the children of Puerto Rican rural migrants in New York than in San Juan because I assumed that the Puerto Rican children in New York experience greater socioeconomic and cultural stress. Instead, I found that the incidence of stuttering among the children attending the public elementary schools of San Juan was considerably higher than among the Puerto Rican children attending the New York public elementary schools, below the 1 percent level of significance. I discovered during my field experiences and my investigation of the lifeways of the migrants in San Juan and New York that I had not sufficiently taken into account the importance of the difference in the dominant values of Puerto Rico and the United States, and the immediate and long-term benefits to the migrants of acculturation in New York.

Stuttering and Nonstuttering Societies

The United States and Puerto Rico share the cultural values and patterns of both the stuttering and the nonstuttering societies discussed earlier, but the two countries differ significantly in the degree to which they share these values.

In their social goals—the achievement of power, prestige, and rank by the accumulation of material property and honorifics—Americans unequivocally resemble the people of the stuttering societies. Striving, competitiveness, aggressiveness are the primary values of the United States and of the stuttering cultures. But as these traits no longer lead so readily to the foremost objective of upward mobility, the counterthemes of security and stability, goals of the nonstuttering societies, have emerged as dominant values of most members of the American working classes, as well as large segments of the middle class.

On the one hand, the Protestant (ethic) reflects the continuing importance of individualism, and on the other, the values of cooperation and community. Community cooperation, characteristic of the nonstuttering cultures, has always been a strong countertheme in the United States, expressed by the abundance of voluntary associations devoted to improving the lot of the individual and the lives of the unfortunate. In addition, Utopian communes, rejecting the dominant values of individualism and materialism, began to emerge as early as 1680, burgeoned during the eighteenth and nineteenth centuries, and are now flourishing in greater numbers than ever before (Kanter 1970:53–57). And to the working classes the cooperative, noncompetitive relationships in the extended family are more important than the nuclear family, as in the nonstuttering societies.

While competitive education is the means of upward mobility in both the United States and the stuttering cultures, American education since the nineteenth century has also had the mission of building a new world in which children could be "freer than we have been—freer from anxiety, freer from guilt and fear, freer from economic constraint and the dictates of expediency" (Mead 1964:172). In the nonstuttering societies the relative freedom of children is also a prominent pattern.

War and violence are institutionalized in the United States, as in the stuttering cultures and, like the stuttering peoples, Americans are intolerant of failure, imperfections, abnormalities, and linguistic variations. But while a high premium is placed on correct speech and speech fluency, freedom of speech is institutionalized and remains a basic value in the United States, as in the nonstuttering societies.

Women and children have always been subordinate in the United States, as in the stuttering societies, but a strong countertheme, since earliest times, is the democratic family, with its emphasis on egalitarian relationships between husband and wife, parents and children. This countertheme, a major value of the nonstuttering cultures, is becoming increasingly dominant in the United States, and is finding expression in the women's liberation and youth movements.

American children were customarily subjected to physical punishment, but during the last twenty-five years the middle class has been resorting more to nonviolent and love-oriented means to discipline and mold the child. Boys are still punished more frequently and severely than girls for the purpose of fostering the "masculine" attributes that are presumed to lead to success, and the boy is pressed to achieve at a young age, as in the stuttering societies. But American youth has a protracted adolescence and is not hurried toward adulthood. As in the nonstuttering cultures, the child's impulses and desires are recognized and honored by more and more adults in all classes.

As the nonstuttering cultures use religion to solve individual problems and to deal with social stress, so Americans have developed a variety of therapeutic and educational measures designed to protect and strengthen individuals exposed to cultural strains:

1) emphasis on a new type of child rearing which takes "self-demand" as the framework for habit formation; 2) the progressive educational movement with its philosophy of letting the child strike its own pace; 3) types of social case work and psychiatry which stress the need for helping the individual work out his own problems and achieve a new integration (Mead 1959:526).

Puerto Rico most resembles the nonstuttering societies in the co-operative relationships of the extended family, which encourages individual achievement only on behalf of the family. Historically, however, cooperation did not extend to the community. The peasants inherited an antisocial individualism from the original settlers and, submerged by their Spanish rulers, were morally and socially passive (G. Lewis 1963:96). Nor is religion a cohesive force, as in the nonstuttering cultures; the great majority of the people have only tenuous ties with Catholicism. Thus community organization and leadership have been weak among Puerto Ricans both on the island and the mainland, and are only now beginning to emerge, particularly on the mainland.

As Puerto Rico industrializes there is an increasing tendency to measure a man by the quantity and quality of his possessions, as in the stuttering cultures. Also, murder and suicide have been frequent responses to shame, again as in the stuttering societies, although war is not institutionalized in Puerto Rico.

Coexisting with modern institutions, the semifeudal social structure in Puerto Rico, with its class stratification and explicit subordination of women and children, most clearly resembles the high-incidence stuttering society of Japan. Puerto Rican culture has few institutionalized therapeutic devices or social outlets for either women or children, and emotional disturbances and suicide have been particularly high among young Puerto Ricans, as among young Japanese. In both cultures a very sharp discontinuity is created by the repression of children after initial indulgence and warmth toward babies.

Although the Puerto Rican extended family and the Spiritualist mediums deal effectively with physical and mental illness, the culture as a whole, like the stuttering societies, has little tolerance for physical and mental abnormalities and for such linguistic deviance as stuttering.

The Puerto Rican value of respect results in parental discouragement of the child's language development and great restraints on his verbal freedom. By contrast, children in the nonstuttering societies have great freedom of speech and are permitted to use verbal aggression and linguistic variations.

In sum, the United States resembles the stuttering cultures in many of its social goals, such as the acquisition of power, rank, prestige, and material possessions; in many of its dominant values, such as individualism, striving, aggressiveness, competitiveness; in its institutions of war and violence; in its intolerance of failure and abnormalties. But it resembles the nonstuttering societies in its emphasis upon community cooperation and voluntary association for social goals; in the noncompetitive extended family relationships, particularly among blue-collar workers; in the egalitarian direction of conjugal and generational roles; in the prevalence of individual and group therapeutic measures and social movements for the mitigation of cultural stress; and in the freedom of speech, verbal aggressiveness, and ego development permitted children.

Puerto Rico resembles the stuttering societies in its new social goals, its use of murder and suicide as responses to shame, the lack of outlets to relieve cultural stress, the subordination of women and children, the intolerance of mental and physical deviations, the severe discontinuities in its child-rearing practices, and the constriction of the child, especially in the realm of speech. It resembles the nonstuttering cultures in the close, cooperative relationships among members of the extended family, the lack of emphasis on individual achievement, and in its indulgence of infants.

Although the cultural patterns of both the United States and Puerto Rico resemble those of the stuttering societies in a number of ways, clearly the values of the United States resemble those of the nonstuttering societies in many more aspects than do the values of Puerto Rico.

Stuttering Incidence and Sociocultural Stress

There is no doubt that the acculturation of the Puerto Rican rural migrants in New York is more immediately stressful than their gradual urbanization in San Juan. Not only are the culture, language, and climate unfamiliar in New York, but rapid acculturation is demanded, racial prejudice and ethnic discrimination are overt and widespread, the Puerto Rican community is dispersed, and many migrants are isolated from the extended family.

On the other hand, the migrants have available resources in New York that are absent in San Juan: the Migration Division of the Commonwealth Department of Labor; Puerto Rican organizations like Aspira that attempt to improve the conditions of the migrants and integrate the Puerto Rican community into the larger society; religious organizations that provide economic assistance and aid grass-roots groups struggling for socioeconomic and political benefits; hometown associations that provide help and recreation and reduce the impact of migration.

The work skills and knowledge of the English language which the migrants acquire in New York contribute to their greater lifetime income, whether they remain on the mainland or return to the island. With income on the mainland approximately double the island income, and welfare assistance at least ten times greater in New York than in San Juan, malnutrition and undernourishment are far less prevalent and physical health is considerably better than in San Juan. The superior medical facilities in New York also lead to better physical and mental health, despite the class arrogance and ethnocentrism of many American medical practitioners and their ignorance of Puerto Rican culture and the Spanish language. In addition, the most decrepit tenements in New York constitute a much lower health hazard than the shantytowns of San Juan.

The New York City school system has instituted many more programs to help Puerto Ricans learn English and acculturate to the mainland than it did for the earlier immigrants, but compensatory education has not been very effective in raising the relatively low achievement level of Puerto Rican children. Nevertheless, the migrants, notably the females, do acquire far more education than in San Juan, and the second generation especially are much more upwardly mobile in New York.

The greater participation of the migrants in economic and political activities in New York than in San Juan, and the "politicalization" of the second generation link many more of the migrants and their children to the larger society in New York, with proportionately fewer in the culture of poverty than in San Juan. Interethnic hostility and competition are partially balanced by interethnic accommodation and collaboration. Puerto Rican identity is finally becoming stronger, and the Puerto Rican community is becoming more cohesive as white Puerto Ricans in New York assert their bilingualism and biculturalism and the darker skinned also acknowledge their African heritage.

Initially family stresses are more intense in New York because of the sharper collision between traditional and modern values, but the demand for rapid acculturation may in the long run be beneficial. In describing the social transformation of the Manus people of the Admiralty Islands,

Margaret Mead (1961b) concluded "that a people who choose to practice new cultural forms will ride the transition more easily if they make all the changes at once," instead of slowly and partially. Although the rapid revision of Puerto Rican conjugal and generational roles creates very severe strains in the family, once the new roles are acquired in New York they are more functional for upward mobility, the goal of the migrants in both cities, than the slow, gradual, partial changes that take place in San Juan.

Thus, although the sociocultural stresses following migration are initially greater in New York, the immediate and long-range economic gains and the long-range sociocultural benefits appear to be far greater for the migrants in New York than in San Juan. These findings, together with the greater concordance between the values of the United States and the nonstuttering societies than between the values of Puerto Rico and these societies, accord with the significantly lower incidence of stuttering in New York, 0.84 percent, than in San Juan, 1.50 percent. The higher incidence in San Juan accords with the "significant trend" for stuttering children to come from families in which the "degree of undesirable social pathology" is greater than in any other segment of the population (Andrews and Harris 1964:30). This "trend" appeared in Newcastle-upon-Tyne, England, and in the several studies (discussed in Chapter 3) which show the much higher stuttering incidence among socioeconomically deprived black than white children throughout the United States.

The much higher stuttering incidence among Puerto Rican boys than girls in New York, 1.44 to 0.23 percent, a ratio of 6:1, appears to reflect the lesser economic adjustment and role revision, as well as the poorer mental health, of Puerto Rican males than females.

The disparity between male and female stuttering incidence in New York is double the disparity between male and female stuttering incidence in San Juan, 2.17 to 0.76 percent, a ratio of about 3:1. The greater sex disparity in New York than in San Juan derives from the same factors that produce the greater disparity between white boys and girls than between black boys and girls in the United States.

Goldman found that the stuttering ratio in black patrifocal families approximated the expected male-female ratio in the United States, and the difference between male and female stuttering incidence was much less in black matrifocal than in patrifocal families. This reflected the increased pressures on the male and decreased pressures on the female in the patrifocal family and the decreased pressures on the male and increased pressures on the female in the matrifocal family (R. Goldman 1967:80). The broken home, more typical of the matrifocal family and the consensual union, appears to affect girls more adversely than boys (Rodman 1968:758). Since the matrifocal family is more prevalent among blacks than among whites, the significantly higher stuttering rate for black females than for white females also appears to be associated with the heavier burdens for females in the matrifocal family.

The rate of consensual union among Puerto Ricans on the mainland, as represented by the migrants who return to Puerto Rico, is less than half the rate of consensual unions in Puerto Rico. It is noteworthy that the stuttering incidence in New York is almost half that in San Juan, and that the male-female disparity in New York is about double that in San Juan. Thus stuttering not only decreases for both sexes with the decrease of the matrifocal family (which is associated with the consensual union) and the increase of the patrifocal family, but decreases much more for girls than for boys under such circumstances. Since in a patriarchal culture the patrifocal family is the norm, it tends to be more stable and less brittle than the matrifocal family.

The lower male incidence in New York than in San Juan, 2.17 to 1.44 percent, or a ratio of 1.5:1, appears to result from the benefits that accrue to the boys when their parents begin to acculturate to the mainland. The more acculturated migrants in New York tend to punish their sons less severely than in San Juan, are less authoritarian, and equalize demonstrations of affection toward boys and girls. Sexual stereotypes, which require the boy to be aggressive and *macho,* are less operative in New York, where the Puerto Rican boy is permitted a more idiosyncratic development. The acculturated adult male is better integrated into the family and presents a more positive role model for his son. The more acculturated male learns to channel aggression in political and economic, not just *macho,* activities. As education and economic opportunity increase, he also integrates more successfully into the larger society. The second-generation male is less equivocal about color, race, and ethnic origin than either his parents or Puerto Ricans on the island, and it is in New York that his ethnic and racial identity is strengthened as he fights for bilingualism, biculturalism and racial equality.

The much higher incidence of stuttering among females in San Juan than in New York, 0.76 to 0.23 percent, or a ratio of about 3:1, not only reflects greater stresses for the female when the matrifocal family and consensual union prevail, but also the far less satisfactory role and status for the girls in San Juan than in New York. With the model of greater freedom and independence for women in New York, and the considerably greater educational and economic opportunities, the Puerto Rican woman has been notably successful in her struggle against subordination, restriction, and role segregation. It is noteworthy that the difference between female stuttering in the two cities is much greater than the difference between male stuttering, attesting to the more far-reaching role revisions among Puerto Rican females than males in New York.

Inferences from the Study

The prevalence of stuttering or the lack of stuttering appears to depend partially on the dominant values of a culture, including its attitudes toward language. The difference in values between the mainland and the island accounts, to an important extent, for the differences in stuttering incidence between the public elementary school children in San Juan and the Puerto Rican children attending the New York City elementary schools.

The findings in this study indicate that, contrary to the Sapir-Whorf hypothesis, it is cultural values, arising out of the lifeways of a society, that determine the purposes of language, the mode of language behavior, and the methods of language teaching. Once in existence, the language patterns reinforce and perpetuate the world view of the culture, but this is a secondary, not a primary, phenomenon. And when the world view changes with changes in the social structures and institutions, the language patterns change to correspond.

Language patterns that constitute assets in one type of society may be disabilities in another type. A Puerto Rican child who is enculturated by the traditional meaning of the word *respeto* may be handicapped for functioning in an industrial society. Although the patterns of behavior symbolized by *respeto* guarantee the individual a form of dignity in Puerto Rico, the word is the symbol for the superordinate and subordinate relationships between the state and the people, the Church and the people, employers and employees, husbands and wives, parents and children. As Puerto Rico changes from a semifeudal, stratified, agricultural society, *respeto* loses its traditional connotations and begins to symbolize the new emerging relationships between the individual and the institutions. *Respeto* has a different connotation in a democratic, industrialized, urban society than in a feudal agricultural society, regardless of the particular language spoken.

The varying rates of stuttering in the several social classes appear to derive from both cultural and socioeconomic factors. I infer that in a relatively open, competitive society the incidence of stuttering will be highest in those strata where the individual is deprived of upward mobility by such social barriers as race, ethnicity, and religion. The stuttering rates among such classes will correlate directly with the degree of discrimination. The stuttering rates will also parallel the rates of homicide, suicide, mental illness, alcoholism, drug addiction, and juvenile delinquency.

The male-female disparity in stuttering incidence appears to derive from the differences between male and female roles and the structure and status of the family in a society. In a patriarchal culture, the male monopolizes power and authority, but when such a society is also competitive, the male status must not only be achieved but must constantly be validated. Since the major female role in a patriarchal culture is biological and female status is ascribed, the woman's status is lower than the man's and her goals are circumscribed, but she is under little pressure to achieve the social goals. Thus in a patriarchal society, male stuttering incidence is generally considerably higher than female stuttering incidence. However, if the female role in a patriarchal society is markedly subordinate and restricted, and the woman has few satisfactory outlets of any kind, as in Japan, female stuttering incidence may be as high as male incidence, if not higher.

In a patriarchal culture, the female in the matrifocal family suffers considerable stress both because her responsibilities increase greatly and because her role as household head is regarded as deviant. Thus the incidence of stuttering for females in matrifocal families will be higher than in patrifocal families where the parents are legally married, which is the norm in a patriarchal society.

I infer that in a society in which descent and inheritance are neither patrilineal nor matrilineal, as in some of the Buddhist cultures, and where male and female role and status are equal and depend on individual talent and ability, there will be no disparity between male and female stuttering. In fact, such a society should have no stuttering.

There appears to be no relationship between stuttering and bilingualism. As a variable associated with learning a second language, stuttering appears to be related to the increments or disadvantages which accrue to such learning and to the sociocultural context in which the language is learned. In New York it is Spanish, the native language of the Puerto Rican migrant, which is a source of ambivalence connected with race and ethnicity. Learning English, on the other hand, results in substantial rewards, and has positive social and psychological effects.

From the relationships which appear to exist between stuttering incidence and stress within the cultural and socioeconomic milieus of San Juan and New York City respectively, I draw the following specific inferences.

In a competitive society, which describes itself as "open," stuttering will decrease among children whose parents have the opportunity for upward mobility and who utilize techniques of child rearing which equip the child for successful adult functioning in the culture. Conversely, stuttering will increase among children whose parents are in strata that are deprived of opportunity and also of the techniques which equip the child for successful adult functioning. Thus the stresses on children in the culture of poverty will induce a higher incidence of stuttering than the stresses on children in any other social segment.

But the children of poor parents who are linked to the larger social institutions by economic, political, social, or religious activity will be less susceptible to the stresses that induce stuttering than the children whose parents are isolated from the major institutions. The cohesive, socially integrated community will also have a lower incidence of stuttering than the community characterized by *anomie*.

When racial discrimination prevails in a competitive society that describes itself as "open," the incidence of stuttering will be highest among the children with the darkest color in each social class and ethnic group.

In such a society the incidence of stuttering will be lower among those classes and subcultures which emphasize the values of egalitarianism, independence, initiative, and self-assertion than among those which emphasize subordination, dependence, passivity, and docility.

In a society which places a premium on the values of competition, egalitarianism, independence, and self-assertion, and permits both sexes to cultivate these qualities, there will be no difference between male and female stuttering incidence. But in competitive society, that describes itself as "open," stereotyped, inflexible, segregated sex roles will create stresses that are more conducive to stuttering among both sexes than flexible, desegregated sex roles.

Sharp discontinuities in role learning will increase uncertainties and anxieties that are more conducive to stuttering than smooth, continuous role preparation.

A culture that is intolerant of physical, mental, emotional, and linguistic differences will create stresses that induce stuttering.

A society that provides therapeutic and educational measures that protect and strengthen the individual and the group in their exposure to cultural stress, and organizational structures that can work for social justice, will have a lower incidence of stuttering than one in which such structures are absent.

A culture in which respect for the child is an important value, and which honors children's impulses and desires will have a lower incidence of stuttering than cultures which lack these values. The marked repression of aggression, in conjunction with the use of frequent and severe physical punishment, ridicule, and shame will create stresses in children that induce a higher incidence of stuttering than the limited repression of aggression, in conjunction with the use of verbal guidance and praise to produce desired behavior. The marked constriction of the ego and of language will be conducive to stuttering, whereas the relatively free development of the ego and of language will be conducive to automatic and fluent speech.

Suggestions for Further Research

In order to refine the relationships between stuttering incidence and sociocultural stress, I recommend that the incidence of stuttering be investigated and compared among children and adults in the following categories:

1. Public schools in poverty areas, and middle- and upper-class private schools

2. The several divisions of the blue-collar working class

3. Blue-collar working-class families that are completely self-supporting and those that receive welfare assistance

4. Blue-collar workers who participate in economic, political, social, and religious activities, and those who are socially isolated

5. Various ethnic groups in the same and different socioeconomic classes

6. Various religious groups in the same and different socioeconomic classes

7. Dark-skinned and white-skinned Puerto Ricans in the several socioeconomic classes on the island and on the mainland

8. Dark-skinned and light-skinned blacks in the several classes in the South and North of the United States

9. Sex ratios in stuttering incidence among matrilineal and patrilineal cultures

10. Sex ratios in patrifocal and matrifocal families in patriarchal societies

11. The different grade levels in elementary and junior high schools [the findings in this study do not indicate why stuttering incidence among Puerto Rican children in both San Juan and New York is highest in the fourth grade, and next highest in the first grade].

Such studies should provide explicit data about the cultural and socioeconomic bases of stuttering etiology, as well as a clear "index of culture stress" (Naroll 1959:108) among children. Since indices of culture stress, such as suicide, homicide, alcoholism, mental illness, and the use of witchcraft have been determined for adults in various societies, stuttering incidence as an index of culture stress among children could serve as the basis for early preventive and alleviative social measures.

Bibliography

Adler, Sol
    1961   An Integration of Some Research Studies in Stuttering. *Rehabilitation Literature* 22, February, pp. 34–41 ff.

American Federation of Labor-Congress of Industrial Organization
    1963   *What Everyone Should Know about Government Spending and Full Employment.* Publication No. 53. Washington, D.C.: AFL-CIO.

Anderson, P.
    1966   Making Trouble Is Alinsky's Business. *The New York Times Magazine.* October 9, pp. 28–31 ff.

Andrews, Gavin, and Mary Harris
    1964   *The Syndrome of Stuttering.* London: Spastics Society Medical and Information Unit, in association with William Heinemann Medical Books, Ltd.

Arensberg, Conrad M.
    1961   The Community as Object and as Sample. *American Anthropologist* 63(2): 241–264.

Arsenian, John, and Jean Arsenian
    1948   Tough and Easy Cultures. *Psychiatry* 11: 377–385.

Back, Kurt W.
    1962   *Slums, Projects and People.* Durham, N.C.: Duke University Press.

Bain, Read
    1935   Our Schizoid Culture. *Sociology and Social Research* 19: 266–276.

Baldwin, James
    1962   Letter from a Region of My Mind. *The New Yorker* 38, November 17, pp. 59–144.

Basden, G. T.
    1921   *Among the Ibos of Nigeria.* New York: Barnes and Noble.

Beals, Ralph
    1951   Urbanism, Urbanization, Acculturation. *American Anthropologist* 53: 1–10.

Beckwith, Lillian
    1962   *The Sea for Breakfast.* New York: E. P. Dutton.
    1969   *A Rope—In Case.* New York: E. P. Dutton.

Benedict, Ruth
    1934   *Patterns of Culture*. Boston: Houghton Mifflin.
    1950   Continuities and Discontinuities in Cultural Conditioning. In Clyde
           Kluckhohn and Henry A. Murray (eds.), *Personality in Nature,
           Society and Culture*. New York: Alfred A. Knopf.

Berle, Beatrice B.
    1958   *80 Puerto Rican Families in New York City*. New York: Columbia
           University Press.

Bible
           Exodus 4: 10–17.
           Isaiah 32: 4.
           Mark 7: 32–37.

Bloodstein, Oliver
    1958   Stuttering as an Anticipatory Struggle Reaction. In Jon Eisenson
           (ed.), *Stuttering, A Symposium*. New York: Harper & Brothers.
    1959   *A Handbook on Stuttering for Professional Workers*. Chicago:
           National Society for Crippled Children and Adults.

Bronfenbrenner, Urie
    1958   Socialization and Social Class through Time and Space In E. E.
           Maccoby, T. M. Newcomb and E. L. Hartley (eds.), *Readings in
           Social Psychology*. 3d ed. New York: Henry Holt.

Brown, Myrtle I.
    1961   Changing Maternity Care Patterns in Migrant Puerto Ricans. Un-
           published Ph.D. dissertation, New York University.

Bullen, Adelaide K.
    1945   A Cross-Cultural Approach to the Problem of Stuttering. *Child
           Development* 16: 1–88.   .

Business Week
    1959   Worker Loses His Class Identity. July 11, p. 90.

Caplovitz, David
    1964   The Problems of Blue-Collar Consumers. In Arthur B. Shostak and
           William Gomberg (eds.), *Blue-Collar World*. Englewood Cliffs,
           N. J.: Prentice-Hall.

Caplow, Theodore, Sheldon Stryker, and Samuel E. Wallace
    1964   *The Urban Ambience*. Totowa, N. J.: Bedminster Press.

Casagrande, J. S.
    1964   Comanche Baby Language. In Dell Hymes (ed.), *Language in Cul-
           ture and Society*. New York: Harper & Brothers.

Caudill, William
    1959   Observations on the Cultural Context of Japanese Psychiatry. In
           Marvin K. Opler (ed.), *Culture and Mental Health*. New York:
           Macmillan.

Chenault, Lawrence R.
    1938   *The Puerto Rican Migrant in New York City*. New York: Columbia
           University Press, 1938.

Chesler, Phyllis
1971 Patient and Patriarch: Women in the Psychotherapeutic Relationship. In Vivian Gornick and Barbara K. Moran (eds.), *Woman in Sexist Society*. New York: Basic Books.

Chess, Stella, et al.
1967 Social Class and Child-Rearing Practices. New York: The Authors, November 17. Mimeographed.

Chinoy, Eli
1952 Aspirations of Automobile Workers. *American Journal of Sociology* 57: 453–459.

Cohen, Albert K., and Harold M. Hodges
1963 Characteristics of the Lower Blue-Collar Class. *Social Problems* 10: 303–334.

Coleman, James S., et al.
1966 *Equality of Educational Opportunity*. Washington, D.C.: U.S. Government Printing Office.

Commonwealth of Puerto Rico
1964 *A Summary in Facts & Figures*. New York: Commonwealth of Puerto Rico, Department of Labor, Migration Division.
1966 *The Puerto Rican Child in His Cultural Context*. Barranquitas: Commonwealth of Puerto Rico, Department of Education. Mimeographed.

Davis, Kingsley
1938 Mental Hygiene and the Class Structure. *Psychiatry* 1: 55–65.

Devereux, George, and Edwin M. Loeb
1943 Antagonistic Acculturation. *American Sociological Review* 8: 133–147.

Diaz-Guerrero, R.
1955 Neurosis and the Mexican Family Structure. *American Journal of Psychiatry* 112: 411–417.

Diebold, A. Richard
1965 A Survey of Psycholinguistic Research, 1954–1964. In G. E. Osgood and T. A. Sebeok (eds.), *Psycholinguistics*. Bloomington, Ind.: Indiana University Press.

Dodson, Dan W.
1968 *In Essence*. Compiled by S. N. Pittman. New York: Vantage Press.

Du Bois, Cora
1955 The Dominant Value Profile of American Culture. *American Anthropologist* 57(6): 1232–1239.

Dyer, William O.
1964 Family Reactions to the Father's Job. In Arthur B. Shostak and William Gomberg (eds.), *Blue-Collar World*. Englewood Cliffs, N. J.: Prentice-Hall.

Eisenson, Jon
1966 Observations on the Incidence of Stuttering in a Special Culture. *ASHA*, October, pp. 391–394.

Elkins, Stanley M.
1959   *Slavery*. New York: Grosset and Dunlap.

Erikson, Erik H.
1964   *Insight and Responsibility*. New York: W. W. Norton.

Evans, Adeline L.
1964   A Survey of the Speech and Hearing Problems of the First Three Grades in Selected Negro Schools of Lincoln Parish. Unpublished M.A. thesis, Louisiana State University.

Fantiti, Mario D., and Gerald Weinstein
1968   *The Disadvantaged: Challenge to Education*. New York: Harper & Row.

Ferman, Louis A.
1964   Sociological Perspectives in Unemployment Research. In Arthur R. Shostak and William Gomberg (eds.), *Blue-Collar World*. Englewood Cliffs, N. J.: Prentice-Hall.

Fitzpatrick, Joseph P.
1955   The Integration of Puerto Ricans. *Thought* 30: 402–420.
1960   Puerto Rican Story. *America,* September 3, p. 595.
1966a Intermarriage of Puerto Ricans in New York City. *American Journal of Sociology* 71: 395–406.
1966b The Role of Language as a Factor of Strength for the Puerto Rican Community. In *The Puerto Rican Child in His Cultural Context*. Barranquitas, P. R.: Commonwealth of Puerto Rico, Department of Education.
1968   Puerto Ricans in Perspective: The Meaning of Migration to the Mainland. *International Migration Review* 2(Spring): 7–20.
1969   Educational Experience of the Puerto Rican Community in New York City. New York: The Author. Mimeographed.

Fitzpatrick, Joseph P. and Robert E. Gould
1968   Mental Health Needs of Spanish-Speaking Children in the New York City Area. A Task Force Paper for the Joint Commission on Mental Health for Children. New York: The Authors. Mimeographed.

Fletcher, John M.
1928   *The Problem of Stuttering*. New York: Longmans, Green.

Flexner, Eleanor
1959   *Century of Struggle*. Cambridge, Mass.: Belknap Press.

Foster, George M.
1953   What Is Folk Culture? *American Anthropologist* 55: 159–173.
1960   *Culture and Conquest, America's Spanish Heritage*. Chicago: Quadrangle Books.

Friedlander, Stanley L.
1965   *Labor Migration and Economic Growth*. Cambridge, Mass.: The M.I.T. Press.

Geertz, Hildred
1961   *The Javanese Family*. Glencoe, Ill.: The Free Press.

Gillin, John
1955　Ethos Components in Latin America. *American Anthropologist*
57: 488–500.

Glazer, Nathan
1959　Introduction. In Stanley M. Elkins, *Slavery*. New York: Grosset
and Dunlap.

Glazer, Nathan, and Daniel P. Moynihan
1963　*Beyond the Melting Pot*. Cambridge, Mass.: The M.I.T. Press.

Golden, Harry
1958　*Only in America*. New York: World.

Goldman, Irving
1961　The Kwakiutl of Vancouver Island. In Margaret Mead (ed.),
Cooperation and Competition among Primitive Peoples. Boston:
Beacon Press.

Goldman, Ronald
1967　Cultural Influences in the Sex Ratio in the Incidence of Stuttering.
American Anthropologist 80: 78–81.

Goldschmidt, Walter
1960　The Comparative Study of Values. In Walter Goldschmidt (ed.),
Exploring the Ways of Mankind. New York: Holt, Rinehart and
Winston.

Goode, William
1946　*The Family*. Englewood Cliffs, N. J.: Prentice-Hall.
1963　*World Revolution and Family Patterns*. London: Free Press of
Glencoe.

Goodstein, L. D.
1958　Functional Speech Disorders and Personality: A Survey of the
Research. *Journal of Speech Research* 1: 359–376.

Goodstein, L. D., and W. G. Dahlstrom
1956　MMPI Differences between Parents of Stuttering and Non-
Stuttering Children. *Journal of Consulting Psychology* 20: 365–371.

Gordon, Edmund W., and Adelaide Jablonsky
1968　Compensatory Education in the Equalization of Educational Opportunity: I and II. *Journal of Negro Education* 38: 268–290.

Gordon, Milton M.
1964　*Assimilation in American Life*. New York: Oxford University Press.

Gray, Lois S.
1962　Economic Incentives to Labor Mobility. Unpublished Ph.D. dissertation, Columbia University.

Greenberg, Joseph H.
1960　Some Aspects of Negro-Mohammedan Culture Contact among the
Hausa. In Simon Ottenberg and Phoebe Ottenberg (eds.), *Cultures
and Societies of Africa*. New York: Random House.

Greene, James S.
1935　Treatment of the Stutter-type Personality in a Medical-Social Clinic.
Journal of the American Medical Association 104: 2239–2242.

Grossman, Arnold H.
1967 *The Launching Pad*. New York: Boys Brotherhood Republic.

Gurin, G., J. Veroff, and S. Feld
1960 *Americans View Their Mental Health*. New York: Basic Books.

Gursslin, O. R., R. G. Hunt, and J. L. Roach
1964 Social Class and Mental Health Movement. In Frank Riessman, Jerome Cohen, and Arthur Pearl (eds.), *Mental Health of the Poor*. New York: The Free Press.

Hamilton, Richard F.
1964 The Behavior and Values of Skilled Workers. In Arthur B. Shostak and William Gomberg (eds.), *Blue-Collar World*. Englewood Cliffs, N. J.: Prentice-Hall.

Handel, G., and L. Rainwater
1964 Persistence and Change in Working Class Life Style. In Arthur B. Shostak and William Gomberg (eds.), *Blue-Collar World*. Englewood Cliffs, N. J.: Prentice-Hall.

Handler, M. S.
1968 Women Give View on Sterilization. *The New York Times,* September 1, p. 25.

Handlin, Oscar
1952 *The Uprooted*. Boston: Little, Brown.
1959 *The Newcomers*. Cambridge, Mass.: Harvard University Press.
1963 *The Americans*. Boston: Little, Brown.

Haring, Douglas G.
1948 Aspects of Personal Culture in Japan. In Douglas G. Haring (ed.), *Personal Character and Cultural Milieu*. Syracuse: Syracuse University Press.

Harris, Marvin
1964 *Patterns of Race in the Americas*. New York: Walker.

Haugen, Einar
1961 The Bilingual Individual. In Sol Saporta (ed.), *Psycholinguistics*. New York: Holt, Rinehart and Winston.

Hernández-Alvarez, José
1967 *Return Migration to Puerto Rico*. Population Monograph Series No. 1. Berkeley: University of California, Institute of International Studies.

Hill, Harris
1944a Stuttering: I. A Critical Review and Evaluation of Biochemical Investigations. *Journal of Speech Disorders* 9: 245–261.
1944b Stuttering: II. A Review and Integration of Physiological Data. Ibid 9: 289–327.

Hill, Reuben, J. Mayone Stycos, and Kurt W. Back
1959 *The Family and Population Control*. Chapel Hill: University of North Carolina Press.

Hoffman, Paul
  1968   City's 2nd-Generation Puerto Ricans Rising from Poverty. *The New York Times,* April 23, pp. 49, 57.

Homans, George C.
  1950   *The Human Group.* New York: Harcourt, Brace.

Honigmann, John J.
  1967   *Personality in Culture.* New York: Harper & Row.

Horwitz, Julius
  1969   A Portrait of New York's Welfare Population. *The New York Times Magazine,* January 26, pp. 22–54.

Hunt, James
  1861   *Stammering and Stuttering.* London: Longmans.

Hurvitz, Nathan
  1964   Marital Strain in the Blue-Collar Family. In Arthur B. Shostak and William Gomberg (eds.), *Blue-Collar World.* Englewood Cliffs, N. J.: Prentice-Hall.

Icken, Helen M.
  1962   From Shanty Town to Public Housing, A Comparison of Family Structure in Two Urban Neighborhoods in Puerto Rico. Unpublished Ph.D. dissertation, Columbia University.

Jarecki, Henry G.
  1961   Maternal Attitudes toward Child Rearing. *Archives of General Psychiatry* 4: 340–355.

Johnson, Wendell
  1944   The Indians Have No Word for It. *Quarterly Journal of Speech* 30: 330–337.
  1956   *Stuttering in Children and Adults.* Minneapolis: University of Minnesota Press.
  1958   Introduction: The Six Men and the Stuttering. In Jon Eisenson (ed.), *Stuttering, A Symposium.* New York: Harper & Brothers.
  1959   *The Onset of Stuttering.* Minneapolis: University of Minnesota Press.
  1967   *Speech Handicapped School Children.* 3rd ed. New York: Harper & Row.

Kanter, Rosabeth Moss
  1970   Communes. *Psychology Today,* July, pp. 53–57.

Kantrowitz, Nathan
  1968   Social Mobility of Puerto Ricans. *International Migration Review* 2(Spring): 53–72.

Karlin, Isaac W., David Karlin, and Louise Gurren
  1965   *Development and Disorders of Speech in Childhood.* Springfield, Ill.: Charles C. Thomas.

Keesing, Felix M.
  1959   *Cultural Anthropology.* New York: Rinehart.

Kennedy, Ruby Jo Reeves
  1944 Single or Triple Melting Pot: Inter-Marriage Trends in New Haven, 1870–1940. *American Journal of Sociology* XLIX: 331–339.

Kihss, Peter
  1968a Illegitimacy Reported Up Here, Involving One of Every 6 Births. *The New York Times,* July 1, p. 21.
  1968b South's Relief Aid Sends Many North. *The New York Times,* October 14, p. 28.
  1969 Relief Here Tops Nation's Average. *The New York Times,* April 8, p. 38.

Klingbeil, G. M.
  1939 The Historical Background of the Modern Speech Clinic. *Journal of Speech Disorders* 4: 115–132.

Kluckhohn, Clyde
  1965 *Mirror for Man.* Greenwich, Conn: Fawcett Publications.

Kluckhohn, Florence R., and Fred Strodtbeck
  1961 *Variations in Value Orientations.* Evanston, Ill.: Row, Peterson.

Kroeber, Alfred L.
  1960 Yurok Speech Usages. In Stanley Diamond (ed.), *Culture in History.* New York: Columbia University Press.

Landy, David
  1965 *Tropical Childhood.* New York: Harper & Row.

Laski, Harold J.
  1948 *The American Democracy.* New York: Viking Press.

Leavitt, Ruby R.
  1962 Auditory Discrimination of Children with Speech and Reading Problems. Unpublished M. S. thesis, Adelphi College.

Lemert, Edwin M.
  1952 Stuttering among the North Pacific Coastal Indians. *Southwestern Journal of Anthropology* 8: 429–41.
  1953 Some Indians Who Stutter. *Journal of Speech and Hearing Disorders* 18: 168–174.
  1962 Stuttering and Social Structure in Two Pacific Societies. *Journal of Speech and Hearing Disorders* 27: 3–10.

Lenski, Gerhard
  1961 *The Religious Factor.* Garden City, N. Y.: Doubleday.

Lesser, G. S., G. Fifer, and D. H. Clark
  1965 Mental Abilities of Children from Different Class and Cultural Groups. *Monographs of the Society for Research in Child Development* 30(4).

Lewis, Gordon K.
  1963 *Puerto Rico, Freedom and Power in the Caribbean.* New York: MR Press.

Lewis, Oscar
  1965 *La Vida.* New York: Random House.

Linton, Ralph
1940a Acculturation and the Processes of Culture Change. In Ralph Linton (ed.), *Acculturation in Seven American Indian Tribes.* New York: D. Appleton-Century.
1940b The Distinctive Aspects of Acculturation. Ibid.

Lipset, Seymour M.
1967 The Unchanging American Character. In Richard L. Rapson (ed.), *Individualism and Conformity in the American Character.* Lexington, Mass.: D. C. Heath.

Lissner, Will
1968 Jobless Rate High for Puerto Ricans. *The New York Times,* September 30, p. 29.

Loether, Herman J.
1964 The Meaning of Work and Adjustment to Retirement. In Arthur B. Shostak and William Gomberg (eds.), *Blue-Collar World.* Englewood Cliffs, N. J.: Prentice-Hall.

Macisco, John J.
1968 Assimilation of the Puerto Ricans on the Mainland. *International Migration Review* 2(Spring): 21–39.

MacLeish, Kenneth
1970 Scotland's Outer Hebrides. *National Geographic* 140 (5): pp. 676–711.

Maier, Henry W.
1965 The Psychoanalytic Theory of Erik H. Erikson. *Three Theories of Child Development.* New York: Harper & Row.

Malzberg, Benjamin
1950 Mental Disease among Puerto Ricans in New York City, 1949–1951. *Journal of Nervous and Mental Disease* 123: 262–269.

Manners, Robert A.
1956 Tabara: Subcultures of a Tobacco and Mixed Crops Municipality. In Julian H. Steward (ed.), *The People of Puerto Rico.* Urbana: University of Illinois Press.

Marge, Michael
1965 The Gift of Speech. *American Education* 1(10): 23–25.

Martindale, Don
1960 *American Society.* New York: D. Van Nostrand.

Martínez, Juan N.
1957 Attitudes and Concepts of a Group of Puerto Rican Professionals Regarding Mental Illness. Unpublished Ph.D. dissertation, New York University.

Marx, Karl
1964 Economic and Philosophic Manuscripts of 1844. In L. E. Horowitz (ed.), *The New Sociology.* New York: Oxford University Press.

Mason, Leonard
1955 The Characterization of American Culture in Studies of Acculturation. *American Anthropologist* 57(6): 1264–1279.

Mayer, K. B., and S. Goldstein
    1964   Manual Workers as Small Business-Men. In Arthur B. Shostak and William Gomberg (eds.), *Blue-Collar World*. Englewood Cliffs, N. J.: Prentice-Hall.

McCullens, J. C., and W. T. Plant
    1964   Personality and Social Development: Cultural Influences. *Review of Educational Research* 34: 599–610.

McPhee, John
    1969   The Island of the Crofter and the Laird. *The New Yorker*, December 6, 1969, pp. 69–165; December 13, pp. 61–112.

McQuown, Norman A.
    1954   Analysis of the Cultural Content of Language Materials. In Harry Hoijer (ed.), *Language in Culture*. Chicago: University of Chicago Press.

Mead, Margaret
    1930   *Growing Up in New Guinea*. New York: William Morrow.
    1942   *And Keep Your Powder Dry*. Ibid.
    1959   The Implications of Culture Change for Personality Development. In Morton W. Fried (ed.), *Readings in Anthropology, II*. New York: Thomas Y. Crowell.
    1961a   Interpretive Statement. In Margaret Mead (ed.), *Cooperation and Competition among Primitive Peoples*. Boston: Beacon Press.
    1961b   *New Lives for Old: Cultural Transformation—Manus, 1928–1953*. New York: Mentor Books.
    1964   Educational Emphases in Perspective. In *Anthropology, A Human Science*. New York: D. Van Nostrand.

Meadows, Paul
    1964   Industrial Man: Another Look at a Familiar Figure. In L. E. Horowitz (ed.), *The New Sociology*. New York: Oxford University Press.

Meier, Dorothy, and Wendell Bell
    1959   Anomia and Differential Access to the Achievement of Life Goals. *American Sociological Review* 24(2): 189–202.

Meltzer, J.
    1953   Relocation of Families Displaced. In C. Woodbury (ed.), *Urban Redevelopment: Problems and Practices*. Chicago: University of Chicago Press.

Mencher, Joan P.
    1958   Child-Rearing and Family Organization among Puerto Ricans in Eastville: *El Barrio de Nueva York*. Unpublished Ph.D. dissertation, Columbia University.

Merton, Robert K.
    1949   *Social Theory and Social Structure*. Chicago: Free Press of Glencoe.

Metraux, Rhoda
    1950   Speech Profiles of the Pre-School Child, 18 to 54 Months. *Journal of Speech and Hearing Disorders* 15: 37–53.

Miller, Daniel R., and Guy E. Swanson
1958 *The Changing American Parent*. New York: John Wiley.

Miller, S. M.
1964a The American Lower Classes: A Typological Approach. In Arthur B. Shostak and William Gomberg (eds.), *Blue-Collar World*. Englewood Cliffs, N. J.: Prentice-Hall.
1964b The New Working Class. Ibid.
1964c The Outlook of Working-Class Youth. Ibid.
1964d Some Thoughts on Reform. Ibid.

Miller, S. M., and Frank Riessman
1964 The Working-Class Subculture: A New View. In Arthur B. Shostak and William Gomberg (eds.), *Blue-Collar World*. Englewood Cliffs, N. J.: Prentice-Hall.

Miller, Walter B.
1958 Lower-Class Culture as a Generating Milieu of Gang Delinquency. *Journal of Social Issues* 14(3): 5–19.

Mills, A. W., and H. Streit
1942 Report of a Speech Survey, Holyoke, Mass. *Journal of Speech Disorders,* July, pp. 161–167.

Mills, C. Wright, Clarence Senior, and Rose K. Goldsen
1950 *The Puerto Rican Journey*. New York: Harper & Brothers.

Mintz, Sidney W.
1953 The Folk-Urban Continuum and the Rural Proletarian Community. *American Journal of Sociology* 59: 136–143.
1956 Canamelar: The Subculture of a Rural Sugar Plantation Proletariat. In Julian H. Steward (ed.), *The People of Puerto Rico*. Urbana: University of Illinois Press.
1960 *Worker in the Cane*. New Haven: Yale University Press.

Minuchin, Salvador, et al.
1967 *Families of the Slums*. New York: Basic Books.

Mizruchi, E. H.
1964 Alienation and Anomie: Theoretical and Empirical Perspectives. In L. E. Horowitz (ed.), *The New Sociology*. New York: Oxford University Press.

Mooney, Richard E.
1968 Parley on Jobs for Puerto Ricans Cites 'Frustration and Despair.' *The New York Times,* May 22, p. 94.

Morgenstern, John J.
1953 Psychological and Social Factors in Children's Stammering. Unpublished Ph.D. dissertation, University of Edinburgh.
1956 Socioeconomic Factors in Stuttering. *Journal of Speech and Hearing Disorders* 21: 25–33.

Mussen, Paul
1966 A Study of Rural Puerto Rican Boys from Agricultural and Factory Families. In *The Puerto Rican Child in His Cultural Context*. Barranquitas: Commonwealth of Puerto Rico, Department of Education.

Naroll, Raoul
  1959   A Tentative Index of Culture Stress. *International Journal of Social Psychiatry* 5: 105–116.

Neely, Margaret M.
  1960   An Investigation of the Incidence of Stuttering among Elementary School Children in the Parochial Schools of Orleans Parish. Unpublished M.A. thesis, Tulane University.

New York City, Board of Education
  1958   *The Puerto Rican Study, 1953–1957.* Brooklyn, N. Y.: Board of Education, City of New York.
  1963   *Special Census of School Population.* Ibid.

The New York Times
  1968   March 26, October 14, November 14, December 25.
  1969   January 19.

Norbeck, Edward, and George de Vos
  1961   Japan. In Francis L. K. Hsu (ed.), *Psychological Anthropology.* Homewood, Ill.: Dorsey Press.

Opler, Marvin K.
  1940   The Southern Ute of Colorado. In Ralph Linton (ed.), *Acculturation in Seven American Indian Tribes.* New York: D. Appleton-Century.
  1959   Dream Analysis in Ute Indian Therapy. In Marvin K. Opler (ed.), *Culture and Mental Health.* New York: Macmillan.

Opler, Morris E.
  1945   Themes as Dynamic Forces in Culture. *American Journal of Sociology* 51(3): 198–201.

Ottenberg, Phoebe
  1959   The Changing Economic Position of Women among the Afikpo Ibo. William R. Bascomb and Melville J. Herskovits. *Continuity and Change in African Cultures.* Chicago: University of Chicago Press.

Ottenberg, Simon
  1959   Ibo Receptivity to Change. Ibid.

Padilla-Seda, Elena
  1956   Nocora: The Subculture of Workers on a Government-Owned Sugar Plantation. In Julian H. Steward (ed.), *The People of Puerto Rico.* Urbana: University of Illinois Press.
  1958   *Up from Puerto Rico.* New York: Columbia University Press.

Patterson, James M.
  1964   Marketing and Working-Class Family. In Arthur B. Shostak and William Gomberg (eds.), *Blue-Collar World.* Englewood Cliffs, N. J.: Prentice-Hall.

Perloff, Harvey S.
  1950   *Puerto Rico's Economic Future.* Chicago: University of Chicago Press.

Pettit, George A.
  1946   *Primitive Education in North America.* Berkeley: University of California Press.

Potter, David M.
1958 *People of Plenty*. Chicago: University of Chicago Press.

Purcell, Theodore V.
1964 The Hopes of Negro Workers for Their Children. In Arthur B. Shostak and William Gomberg (eds.), *Blue-Collar World*. Englewood Cliffs, N. J.: Prentice-Hall.

Rainwater, L., and Handel, G.
1964 Changing Family Roles in the Working Class. Ibid.

Redfield, Robert
1941 *The Folk Culture of Yucatan*. Chicago: University of Chicago Press.

Redfield, Robert, Ralph Linton, and Melville J. Herskovits
1936 A Memorandum for the Study of Acculturation. *American Anthropologist* 38 (1): 149–152.

Riesman, David
1950 *The Lonely Crowd*. New Haven: Yale University Press.

Reissman, Frank
1962 *The Culturally Deprived Child*. New York: Harper & Row.

Rivers, Paula
1964 A Comparative Study of the Number of Speech Defectives among Ethnic Groups in the New York City Elementary and Junior High Schools. Unpublished M.S. thesis, Brooklyn College.

Rodman, Hyman
1964 Middle-Class Misconceptions about Lower-Class Families. In Arthur B. Shostak and William Gomberg (eds.), *Blue-Collar World*. Englewood Cliffs, N. J.: Prentice-Hall.

Rogler, Lloyd H., and August B. Hollingshead
1965 *Trapped: Families and Schizophrenia*. New York: John Wiley.

Rosenblatt, Daniel, and Edward A. Suchman
1964 The Under-Utilization of Medical-Care Services by Blue-Collarites. In Arthur B. Shostak and William Gomberg (eds.), *Blue-Collar World*. Englewood Cliffs, N. J.: Prentice-Hall.

Rosengren, William R.
1964 Social Class and Becoming "Ill." Ibid.

Rothenberg, Albert
1964 Puerto Rico and Aggression. *American Journal of Psychiatry* 120: 926–970.

Sapir, Edward
1921 *Language*. New York: Harcourt, Brace.
1959 Abnormal Types of Speech in Nootka. In David G. Mandelbaum (ed.), *Selected Writings of Edward Sapir in Language, Culture and Personality*. Berkeley: University of California Press.
1966a Language. In David G. Mandelbaum (ed.), *Culture, Language and Personality*. Berkeley: University of California Press.
1966b The Status of Linguistics as a Science. Ibid.
1966c Culture, Genuine and Spurious. Ibid.

Schuell, Hildred M.
  1946   Sex Differences in Relation to Stuttering. Part I. *Journal of Speech Disorders,* November, pp. 277–298.
  1947   Sex Differences in Relation to Stuttering. Part II. Ibid., December, 23–38.

Schuetz, Alfred
  1960   The Stranger. In Maurice R. Stein, Arthur J. Vidich, and David M. White (eds.), *Identity and Anxiety.* New York: The Free Press.

Schwartz, M., and O. Henderson
  1964   The Culture of Unemployment: Some Notes on Negro Children. In Arthur B. Shostak and William Gomberg (eds.), *Blue-Collar World.* Englewood Cliffs, N. J.: Prentice-Hall.

Seda-Bonilla, Edwin
  1958   The Normative Patterns of the Puerto Rican Family in Various Situational Contexts. Unpublished Ph.D. dissertation, Columbia University.
  1966   Social Structure and Race Relations. In S. W. Webster (ed.), *Knowing the Disadvantaged.* San Francisco: Chandler.

Senior, Clarence
  1961   *The Puerto Ricans.* Chicago: Quadrangle Books.
  1968   The Puerto Ricans in New York: A Progress Note. *International Migration Review* 2(Spring): 73–79.

Sexton, Patricia
  1964   Wife of the "Happy Worker." In Arthur B. Shostak and William Gomberg (eds.), *Blue-Collar World.* Englewood Cliffs, N. J.: Prentice-Hall.
  1965   *Spanish Harlem.* New York: Harper & Row.

Shakespeare, William
          As You Like It, III, ii, 198.

Sheehan, Joseph
  1958   Conflict Theory of Stuttering. In Jon Eisenson (ed.), *Stuttering, A Symposium.* New York: Harper & Brothers.

Shostak, Arthur B., and William Gomberg (eds.)
  1964   *Blue-Collar World.* Englewood Cliffs, N. J.: Prentice-Hall.

Sikkema, Mildred
  1948   Observations on Japanese Early Child Training. In Douglas C. Haring (ed.), *Personal Character and Cultural Milieu.* Syracuse: Syracuse University Press.

Smith, Alfred G. (ed.)
  1966   *Communication and Culture.* New York: Holt, Rinehart and Winston.

Smith, Mary
  1954   *Baba of Karo.* London: Faber & Faber.

Snidecor, John C.
  1947   Why the Indian Does Not Stutter. *Quarterly Journal of Speech* 33: 493–495.

Social Science Research Council
1954 Acculturation: An Explanatory Formulation. *American Anthropologist* 56: 973–1002.

Spencer, Robert F. et al.
1965 *The Native Americans.* New York: Harper & Row.

Spinrad, William
1964 Blue-Collar Workers as City and Suburban Residents—Effects on Union Membership. In Arthur B. Shostak and William Gomberg (eds.), *Blue-Collar World.* Englewood Cliffs, N. J.: Prentice-Hall.

Spock, Benjamin
1957 *Baby and Child Care.* New York: Pocket Books.

Srole, Leo, et al.
1962 *Mental Health in the Metropolis: The Midtown Manhattan Study.* New York: McGraw-Hill.

Stamler, Rose
1964 Acculturation and Negro Blue-Collar Workers. In Arthur B. Shostak and William Gomberg (eds.), *Blue-Collar World.* Englewood Cliffs, N. J.: Prentice-Hall.

Stanton, Hazel
1966 Unity and Diversity in Puerto Rican Culture. In *The Puerto Rican Child in His Culture Context.* Barranquitas: Commonwealth of Puerto Rico, Department of Education.

Steward, Julian H. (ed.)
1956 *The People of Puerto Rico.* Urbana: University of Illinois Press.

Stewart, Joseph L.
1960 The Problem of Stuttering in Certain North American Indian Societies. *Journal of Speech and Hearing Disorders.* Monograph Supplement 6.

Sunley, Robert
1955 Early Nineteenth-Century American Literature on Child Rearing. In Margaret Mead and Martha Wolfenstein (eds.), *Childhood in Contemporary Cultures.* Chicago: University of Chicago Press.

Swados, Harvey
1960 The Myth of the Happy Worker. In Maurice R. Stein, Arthur J. Vidich, and David M. White (eds.), *Identity and Anxiety.* New York: The Free Press.

Tawney, Richard H.
1958 Economic Virtues and Prescriptions for Poverty. In H. D. Stein and R. A. Cloward (eds.), *Social Perspectives on Behavior.* New York: Free Press of Glencoe.

Tocqueville, Alexis de
1956 *Democracy in America.* Richard D. Heffner (ed.). New York: The New American Library of World Literature.

Travis, Lee E.
1957 *Handbook of Speech Pathology.* New York: Appleton-Century-Crofts.

Travis, Lee E., Wendell Johnson, and Jayne Shover
1937   The Relation of Bilingualism to Stuttering. *Journal of Speech Disorders* 2: 185–189.

Tumin, Melvin M. and Arnold Feldman
1961   *Social Class and Social Change in Puerto Rico.* Princeton, N. J.: Princeton University Press.

Turner, Frederick Jackson
1920   *The Frontier in American History.* New York: Holt, Rinehart and Winston.

Turner, Nancy
1971   Matrifocality in Indonesia and among Black Americans. Paper presented at the Annual Meeting of the American Anthropological Association, November.

Uchendu, Victor C.
1965   *The Igbo of Southeast Nigeria.* New York: Holt, Rinehart and Winston.

Underwood, Benton J., et al.
1954   *Elementary Statistics.* New York: Appleton-Century-Crofts.

United States Department of Labor, Bureau of Labor Statistics
1968   *Labor Force Experience of the Puerto Rican Worker.* Regional Report No. 9. New York: United States Department of Labor, Bureau of Labor Statistics (June).

Van Riper, Charles
1954   *Speech Correction: Principles and Methods.* 3rd ed. New York: Prentice-Hall.

Vernon, Glenn M.
1964   Religion and the Blue-Collarite. In Arthur B. Shostak and William Gomberg (eds.), *Blue-Collar World.* Englewood Cliffs, N. J.: Prentice-Hall.

Waddle, Elsie L.
1934   A Comparison of the Speech Defects of Colored and White Children. Unpublished M.A. thesis, University of Iowa.

Wakefield, Daniel
1959   *Island in the City.* Boston: Houghton Mifflin.

Wallace, Karl, et al.
1954   *A History of Speech Education in America.* New York: Appleton-Century-Crofts.

Waugh, Alec
1956   Rivals: "New York Is Unique." *The New York Times Magazine,* April 29, pp. 24–70.

Weber, Max
1960   The Ethical Basis of Modern Capitalism. In Walter Goldschmidt (ed.), *Exploring the Ways of Mankind.* New York: Holt, Rinehart and Winston.

Weinreich, Uriel
1961   Languages in Contact. In Sol Saporta (ed.), *Psycholinguistics*. New York: Holt, Rinehart and Winston.

Weissman, Julius
1966   An Exploratory Study of Communication Patterns of Lower-Class Negro and Puerto Rican Mothers and Pre-School Children. Unpublished Ed.D. dissertation, Columbia University.

Whorf, Benjamin S.
1964   Science and Linguistics. In John Carroll (ed.), *Language and Thought*. Englewood Cliffs, N. J.: Prentice-Hall.

Wiener, Norbert
1954   *The Human Use of Human Beings*. Boston: Houghton Mifflin.

Will, Robert E., and Harold G. Vatter (eds.)
1965   *Poverty in Affluence*. New York: Harcourt, Brace & World.

William, Eric
1945   Race Relations in Puerto Rico and the Virgin Islands. *Foreign Affairs* 23: 308–317.

Winthrop, John
1961   A Model of Christian Charity. In Oscar Handlin (ed.), *American Principles and Issues*. New York: Holt, Rinehart and Winston.

Wolf, Eric R.
1956   San Jose: Subcultures of a "Traditional" Coffee Municipality. In Julian Steward (ed.), *The People of Puerto Rico*. Urbana: University of Illinois Press.

Wolf, Kathleen L.
1952   Growing Up and Its Price in Three Puerto Rican Subcultures. *Psychiatry* 15(4): 401–433.

Wolfe, Thomas
1939   *The Web and the Rock*. New York: Harper & Brothers.

Wolfenstein, Martha
1955   Fun Morality: An Analysis of Recent American Child-Training Literature. In Margaret Mead and Martha Wolfenstein (eds.), *Childhood in Contemporary Cultures*. Chicago: University of Chicago Press.

Wright, Louis B.
1957   *The Cultural Life of the American Colonies*. New York: Harper & Row.

Index